the new Diabetes COOKBOOK

the new Diabetes COOKBOOK

100 MOUTHWATERING, SEASONAL, WHOLE-FOOD RECIPES

Kate Gardner, MS, RD

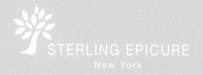

STERLING EPICURE
New York

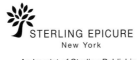

STERLING EPICURE
New York

An Imprint of Sterling Publishing
1166 Avenue of the Americas
New York, NY 10036

ISBN 978-1-4549-1432-7

Distributed in Canada by Sterling Publishing
c/o Canadian Manda Group, 664 Annette Street
Toronto, Ontario, Canada M6S 2C8
Distributed in the United Kingdom by GMC Distribution Services
Castle Place, 166 High Street, Lewes, East Sussex, England BN7 1XU
Distributed in Australia by Capricorn Link (Australia) Pty. Ltd.
P.O. Box 704, Windsor, NSW 2756, Australia

Designed by Christine Heun

For information about custom editions, special sales, and premium and corporate purchases,
please contact Sterling Special Sales at 800-805-5489 or specialsales@sterlingpublishing.com.

Manufactured in China

2 4 6 8 10 9 7 5 3 1

www.sterlingpublishing.com

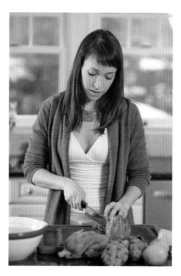

This book is dedicated to my mother for teaching me to cook and nourish myself and to my father for being an ever-willing taster. To my brothers and sister-in-law, who always eat anything (and everything) I prepare and to the rest of my family members for being my biggest fans. Lastly, this book is dedicated to my partner, dishwasher, and photographer, Graham, whose talent and love for both food and photography make everything look delicious.

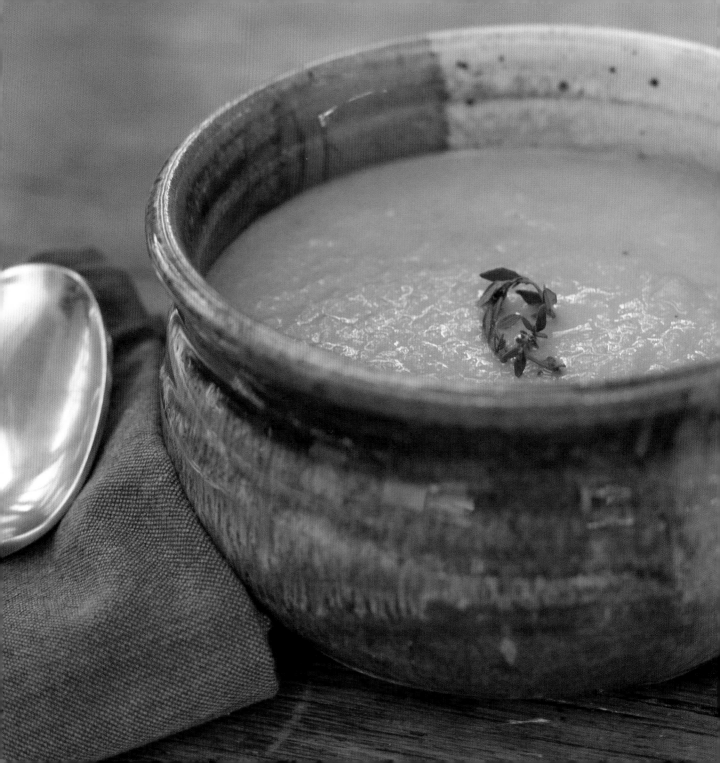

Contents

Foreword

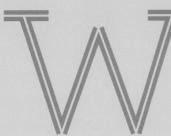hat can I eat? How much should I eat? Should my diet be low-carbohydrate or low-fat? How can I lose weight? These are all common questions, not only of persons with newly diagnosed diabetes mellitus but also of type 1 and type 2 diabetic persons of all ages and duration. Indeed, the American Diabetes Association Clinical Practice guidelines recommend individualized medical nutrition therapy to achieve treatment goals in all persons with pre-diabetes

or diabetes. It is recognized that a variety of eating patterns are acceptable for the diabetes management.

These questions have a greater urgency with the epidemic of diabetes in the United States. In addition, the magnitude of the increase in obesity amplifies this problem. What we eat and how much we eat are not only metabolic issues but also affect heart, lung, liver, and muscle function. Given this importance, healthy eating can be a difficult concept to understand. People want practical solutions to their nutritional questions as part of their overall diabetes care.

Kate Gardner's *The New Diabetes Cookbook* is an important resource to guide people to healthy eating. Not only is proper nutrition understandable, Kate has made healthy eating fun and exciting! Using readily obtainable ingredients, she has created easy-to-prepare diverse and tasty recipes that should satisfy even the most discerning palate. Her recipes have designated portion sizes that will help people to understand how much to eat. She lists carbohydrate, protein, and fat content so that people can understand what they are eating. With her helpful guidance, the transition to healthy eating becomes easier, and less intimidating.

Let Kate Gardner guide you to healthy eating by showing how to prepare appropriate-sized, easy-to-prepare tasty recipes that will improve your meals and overall health.

Stephen G. Rosen, MD
Pennsylvania Hospital
University of Pennsylvania
Philadelphia, PA

Introduction

I was raised in a family where we grew vegetables in our own garden. I found carrots instead of chips in my lunch box, and sugary cereals were served for dessert—not at breakfast. I was fortunate to grow up learning to cook meals from scratch, because that's what my mom did, and what her mom did, and because that was all they could afford. I had no idea I was eating "healthy."

Cooking and eating well with diabetes isn't easy. On top of all the typical challenges to the home cook (time, energy, ingredients on hand, etc.)—there are also worries about carbohydrate content, blood sugar, and making the "right" choices.

I wrote this book because over the many years that I've worked with people who have diabetes, I've heard them say that they are told by nurses and doctors to "Stop eating sugar! Avoid carbohydrates and *no more fruit!*" In two words, my reaction is: *I disagree*.

I've had success helping people with diabetes control their blood sugar while continuing to eat carbohydrate-based foods, *including* fruit and sugars. I believe that eating well with diabetes is about eating whole, unprocessed foods in moderate portions. *Artificial sweeteners and highly processed ingredients have no place in my kitchen—and they should not have a place in yours, either!* I want you to enjoy real butter, real sugar, and real food. You can identify real food just by looking at it. For instance, a chicken is a chicken, not a chicken nugget. And right away, you can recognize a tomato—it doesn't need a box or a label or fancy packaging.

I know this may be a new way of eating and a new way of thinking about food, but controlling diabetes is about learning to eat in a new way. By choosing whole foods when they're in season, you are choosing a more sustainable, more nutritious lifestyle. And that's what it's all about—a healthy lifestyle, where eating healthy begins with cooking.

Being an adventurous cook is simply about building your kitchen confidence—it's about experimenting and failing, followed by experimenting and succeeding. It's about knowing your ingredients and using them to best advantage. None of this is anything more than a learned skill.

Cooking creates both a chemical and an emotional bond with food; it helps you value where ingredients come from and the work it takes to grow, raise, and prepare your meal. It can make you feel happy and responsible for your own well-being, while satisfying the basic need to eat.

Most important, enjoy your food! Make cooking an activity you look forward to and make eating a happy and memorable experience. With this book, eating with diabetes will never be bland or boring again.

Eat well,

Kate Gardner, MS, RD

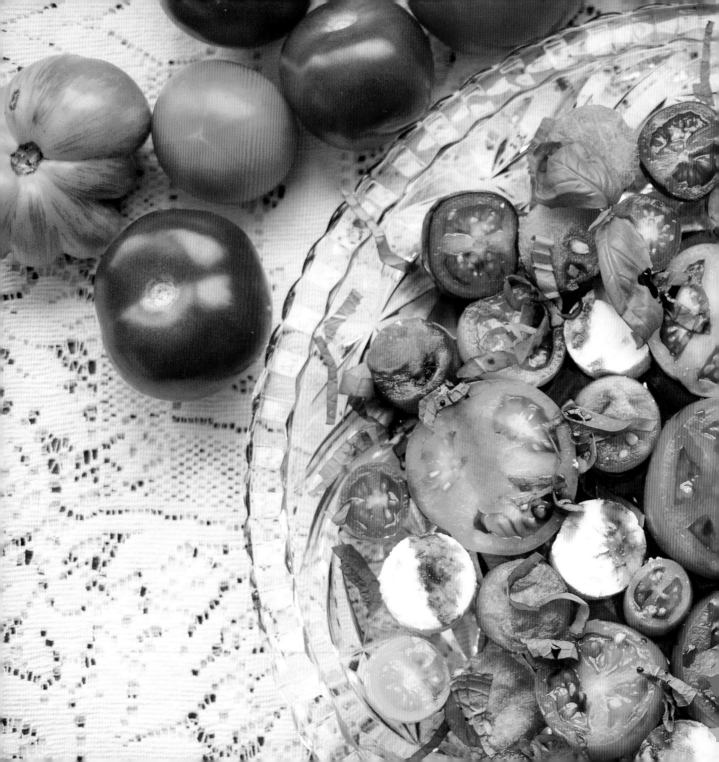

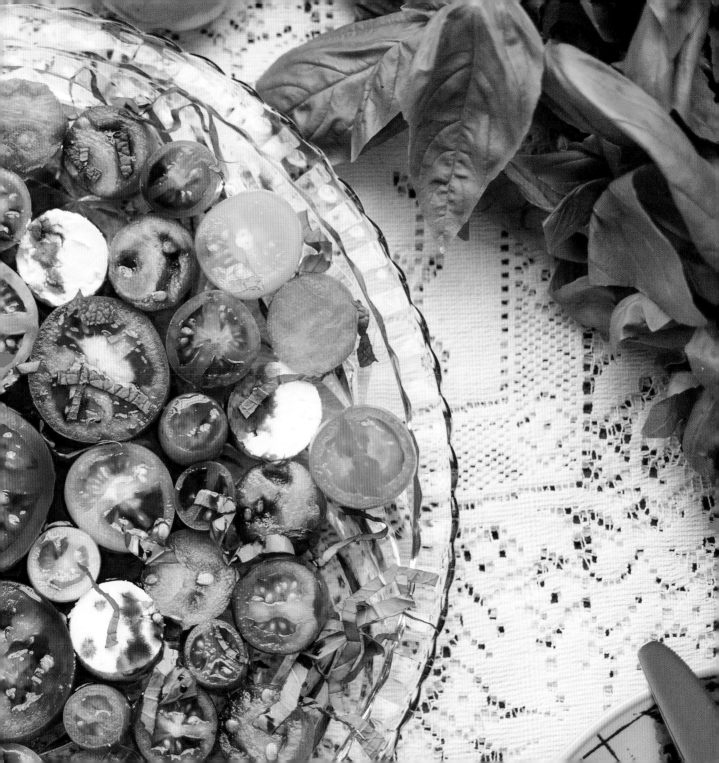

Tips for Using This Book

There are a few critical items for your kitchen that are worth the money, because some will instantly improve your cooking and others will definitely improve your health. Here are my top three choices for must-have items:

1. *Olive oil sprayer*—You can fill one of these handy sprayers with any type of oil you choose. A sprayer helps control how much oil you use and can quickly cut hundreds of calories. While many oils have healthy fat, the calories add up. You can easily control portion size with a sprayer.

2. *Meat thermometer*—I'm proud to say that when I cook meat, it almost always comes out tender and juicy. The reason why I can say that with so much confidence is because I always use a meat thermometer. Not only does it help give you the best results every time, but you don't have to worry about the exact number of minutes it takes to cook a dish. Your oven may not stay at the exact temperature you want and it may circulate air differently than any another oven—so the best cooking time in your oven is probably not the best cooking time in mine. Instead of worrying about how accurate your oven is, cut the hassle, use a meat thermometer and eat delicious food every time you use your oven. See page xvi for a guide on Safe Temperatures for Cooked Food.

3. *Immersion blender*—For many recipes that require a food processor, blender, or hand mixer, you can use an immersion blender. A piece of advice: don't "splurge" on cordless versions; they simply don't have as much power as the ones you plug in, and it's a hassle to make sure they've got enough power for only 2–3 minutes of use. Immersion blenders often come with attachments such as a whip, which makes it versatile, easier to store than a 12-cup food processor, and worth every penny.

What Are the Nutrition Notes?

You'll notice a section in each recipe that highlights a fact or provides extra information about the dish or its ingredients. I've included these Nutrition Notes to arm you with information to make healthier choices in the future. You've picked up the book—you *want* to eat better and I want to help you do that!

Some Nutrition Notes are fun facts or bust food myths, others are written to introduce you to a new food, but almost all of them share information about *why* I've chosen a particular ingredient or cooking method.

How to Create Meals

You'll find that crafting meals with this book will be easy and the food will taste great. Many people with diabetes should have between 45–60 grams of carbohydrate per meal (that's 3–4 carbohydrate exchanges, since 1 exchange = 15 grams of carbohydrates). If you're not sure how much you should have, talk to a dietitian. Better awareness of how much carbohydrate you're eating will mean better blood sugar control, better balance with medications, and better weight management.

As you know, carbohydrates are found in starch (like bread and pasta), fruit, milk, and starchy vegetables (like corn and peas). The amount of carbohydrate you eat will directly affect how much your blood sugar increases. Of course, there are other factors, like fiber, which has an effect—another reason why choosing fiber-rich whole foods is better for you.

In this book, no recipe has more than 45 grams of carbohydrate. So if 45 grams is your maximum, you can select your meal's composition based on that—and you'll have plenty of good options.

Menu Ideas

If you want a healthy, balanced three-course meal, your menu should look like the one at left below. Also shown are practical, healthy menus for a two-course meal and a quick meal.

THREE-COURSE	TWO-COURSE	QUICK MEAL
APPETIZER	**APPETIZER**	**MAIN**
Artichoke Baked Eggs *(10 g)*	Orange-Ginger Tuna Ceviche *(13 g)*	Farmhouse Salad *(41 g)*
MAIN DISH		**DESSERT**
Whole Roasted Trout with Fennel and Sage *(3 g)*	**MAIN DISH**	French Toast Quiche with Strawberries and Basil *(13 g)*
SIDE	Cold Peanut "Noodles" *(30 g)*	
Golden Beet and Zucchini Crisps *(9 g)*		
DESSERT		
Baklava Bundles *(13 g)*		
TOTAL GRAMS OF CARBOHYDRATES	TOTAL GRAMS OF CARBOHYDRATES	TOTAL GRAMS OF CARBOHYDRATES
35	43	54

As you can see, this book provides many ways to combine foods to create a wide choice of meals. To create your own menu—whether it's for lunch or dinner—just add up the number of carbohydrates in each dish you want to make. It's as simple as that!

Each section of the book has recipes that vary in carbohydrate content—except for desserts. As you know, desserts are difficult when you're diabetic because everything sweet has sugar in, it, whether it occurs naturally (as in fresh fruit) or if it's added sugar. I don't like to use artificial sweeteners, so I treat dessert as a special, "once in a while" food. I've tried to give you lots of options here, all of which are controlled for carbohydrate content and can be worked into a three-course meal.

Safe Temperatures for Cooked Food

Leftovers and casseroles   165°F

Ground Meat and Meat Mixtures

Beef, pork, veal, lamb   160°F

Turkey, chicken   165°F

Fresh beef, veal, lamb
Medium rare   145°F
Medium   160°F
Well done   170°F

Poultry

Whole poultry and parts   165°F

Stuffing (cooked alone or in bird)   165°F

Fresh pork
Medium   145°F
Well done   160°F

Ham
Fresh (raw)   145°F
Pre-cooked (to reheat)   140°F

Eggs and Egg Dishes

Eggs: cook until yolks and whites are firm
Egg dishes   160°F

Seafood

Fin fish: 145°F
or flesh is opaque and separates easily

Shrimp, lobster, and crab:
Flesh pearly and opaque

Clams, oysters, and mussels:
Shells open during cooking

Scallops: Mildly white or opaque and firm

Author's Note

AS AN INFORMALLY TAUGHT COOK, I HAVE developed my own style of cooking. It's about eating food that is grown locally by neighbors and friends, perhaps even by farmers, who care as much as you do about how and what you eat.

As a consequence, the recipes in this book are no frills; there's no "fancy" processing and there's nothing fake or artificial. Instead, you'll discover real food that's nutrient rich, hearty, and affordable. You'll also find that shopping for locally grown food and making healthy dishes from scratch also yield meals with a lot of flavor that provide a gratifying sense of fullness (without feeling stuffed). You'll be satisfied, too, by seeing pounds peel away as you get farther away from large portions of highly processed foods that have become so widely available and that have had such a disastrous impact on our waistlines and health.

This book is all about bringing enjoyment back to cooking and eating, while discovering new and sustainable ways to eat responsibly—that is, for your health and for the health of the environment. You'll be amazed by how good the food tastes and how good it makes you feel.

—Kate Gardner, MS, RD

Appetizers, Soups, and Salads

The appetizer course is meant to be a tease—a tempting prelude to the main meal. If you start off with an enticing taste, you will be left wanting more. Since they're small, appetizers can be a little more decadent—like Buffalo Chicken Cigars, which I've served at several dinner parties—and the only reason I keep doing it is because they're in high demand! Appetizers should be foods you shouldn't have a lot of. Instead, think of them as a mild indulgence—like bagel chips or panzanella, two dishes that are frequently touted as off limits to diabetics but are perfectly healthy in starter-size portions.

Reconstructed
Niçoise Salad

Well balanced in texture and flavor, Niçoise salads have a heartiness that other salads lack. However, in the winter and early spring, I prefer hot foods over cold salads, which inspired this delicious warm version.

Serves 4

3 medium red potatoes

½ cup grated cheddar cheese

Salt and freshly ground black pepper

4 tablespoons balsamic vinegar

2 tablespoons Dijon mustard (divided)

3 tablespoons olive oil

½ pound green beans, trimmed

2 cans albacore tuna, packed in water

2 eggs, lightly beaten

⅓ cup grated red onion

⅓ cup panko

2 tablespoons chopped chives

1 tablespoon capers

1 tablespoon dried parsley

1 teaspoon ground coriander

½ teaspoon ground cumin

¼ teaspoon garlic powder

6 cups arugula, chopped

Preheat the oven to 375°F. Using a mandoline, cut the potatoes into 1⁄16-inch-thick slices. Layer the potatoes and cheese in four 6-ounce ramekins and season with salt and pepper. Bake until potatoes are easily pierced with a fork, about 25 minutes.

Meanwhile, whisk together the balsamic vinegar, 1 tablespoon of mustard, 2 tablespoons olive oil, and salt and pepper to taste in a small bowl. Set aside.

Chop half of the green beans into ¾-inch pieces. Finely chop the remaining green beans, uncooked, and set aside.

Drain the tuna fish and squeeze out the excess water. In a medium bowl, gently mix together the tuna, eggs, red onion, panko, chives, 1 tablespoon of mustard, capers, dried parsley, coriander, cumin, and garlic powder. Season to taste with black pepper. Shape the mixture into 4 patties, either by hand or by packing it into a 2-inch round cookie cutter.

Heat a skillet over medium heat and add the remaining 1 tablespoon olive oil. Add the fish cakes and cook until lightly browned on each side. Remove from the heat.

Divide the arugula between 4 plates or bowls. Top with the warm potato cakes, finely chopped green beans, and the fish cakes. Garnish with the longer pieces of green beans and drizzle with some of the balsamic Dijon vinaigrette.

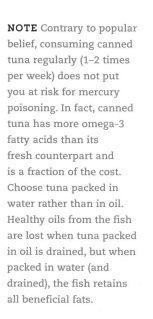

NOTE Contrary to popular belief, consuming canned tuna regularly (1–2 times per week) does not put you at risk for mercury poisoning. In fact, canned tuna has more omega-3 fatty acids than its fresh counterpart and is a fraction of the cost. Choose tuna packed in water rather than in oil. Healthy oils from the fish are lost when tuna packed in oil is drained, but when packed in water (and drained), the fish retains all beneficial fats.

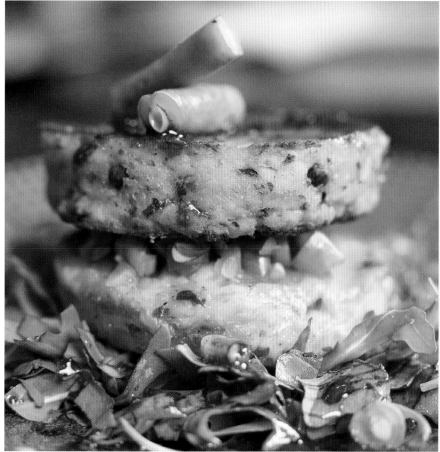

NUTRITION INFORMATION: SERVING SIZE: 1 salad • CALORIES: 360 • CALORIES FROM FAT: 130 • TOTAL FAT: 15 grams • SATURATED FAT: 5 grams • CHOLESTEROL: 135 milligrams • SODIUM: 580 milligrams • TOTAL CARBOHYDRATE: 33 grams • FIBER: 5 grams • PROTEIN: 25 grams

Artichoke
Baked Eggs

Artichokes might be my favorite spring vegetable, but the amount of cleaning and trimming they require is daunting. That's why I think this recipe is great—eating the artichoke from the inside out makes it the easiest, no-hassle artichoke recipe I've ever tried.

Serves 6

2 tablespoons lemon juice

3 cups cold water

3 artichokes

1 tablespoon chopped marjoram

10 green olives, diced

Freshly ground black pepper

⅔ cup nutritional yeast or grated Parmesan

6 eggs

Preheat the oven to 375°F. Fill a bowl with the lemon juice and water. Trim the bottom of an artichoke, pull off the outermost leaves, slice the artichoke in half, and scoop out the inside of the fibrous choke with a spoon. After cleaning each half, place it in the bowl of lemon water to prevent oxidation. Repeat with the remaining artichokes.

Spray a roasting pan lightly with oil and set the artichokes inside, cut side up. Season the artichokes with the marjoram, olives, black pepper, and then sprinkle with the nutritional yeast (or Parmesan). Cover the pan with foil and roast until the artichokes are cooked through and the edges are starting to brown, about 30 minutes. (If you are making this recipe ahead, stop at this step and refrigerate it a few hours or overnight.)

Reduce the oven temperature to 325°F. Uncover the pan and crack an egg into each artichoke half, making sure that it is sitting evenly so that the egg doesn't spill over the side. Bake until the whites are set, about 10 minutes.

Note: An egg will be cracked in the center of each artichoke half, so make sure there is enough space for an egg to fit without spilling out.

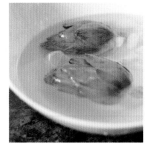

NOTE Nutritional yeast, which is different from brewer's yeast or active dry yeast for baking, is packed with vitamins and minerals. Choose a variety rich in vitamin B_{12}, which can be difficult to find in many vegetarian foods. Nutritional yeast has a rich, cheesy flavor without all the fat.

NUTRITION INFORMATION: SERVING SIZE: ½ artichoke with egg • CALORIES: 160 • CALORIES FROM FAT: 90 • TOTAL FAT: 9 grams • SATURATED FAT: 3 grams • CHOLESTEROL: 190 milligrams • SODIUM: 350 milligrams • TOTAL CARBOHYDRATE: 10 grams • FIBER: 5 grams • PROTEIN: 12 grams

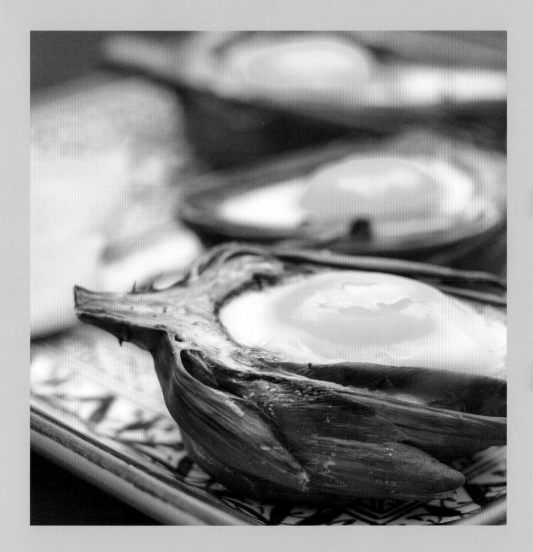

Lemongrass and
Chicken Dumplings

My dumplings are not pretty, they don't have beautiful, even folds—in fact, they're haphazard and a little wonky. But they are tasty. Grated coconut adds enough fat to make these lean chicken dumplings juicy, and the lemongrass balances it with the right amount of acid.

Serves 6

½ pound ground chicken

⅓ cup shredded unsweetened coconut

2 teaspoons sliced jarred lemongrass

2 teaspoons chopped Thai basil

1 teaspoon freshly grated ginger

¼ teaspoon garlic powder

Salt and freshly ground black pepper

30 wonton wrappers

1 egg, lightly beaten with 1 tablespoon water

6 tablespoons low-sodium soy sauce

Mix together the ground chicken, coconut, lemongrass, basil, ginger, and garlic powder. Season to taste with salt and pepper.

Place about 1½ teaspoons of the filling on the middle of a wonton wrapper. Brush the egg wash on the edges of the wrapper and bring the corners together, sealing the dumplings. Repeat with the remaining filling and wrappers.

Set a steamer basket in a wok or a pot, add enough water so that the steamer base sits in the water but the tray sits above it, and bring to a boil. Line the basket with parchment paper, to keep the dumplings from sticking. Working in batches, place dumplings in the basket, cover, and steam until the wrappers are translucent and the filling is cooked through, about 3 minutes. Repeat with the remaining dumplings.

Serve the warm dumplings with low-sodium soy sauce.

NOTE Nasoya purchases domestically grown soy, as well as organic (and non-GMO) products. When you read food labels, aim for processed foods with five ingredients or less—while Nasoya dumpling wrappers have a couple of ingredients, you'll recognize every item on the list as a "real food" ingredient.

NUTRITION INFORMATION: SERVING SIZE: 5 dumplings + 1 tablespoon soy sauce • CALORIES: 190 • CALORIES FROM FAT: 60 • TOTAL FAT: 7 grams • SATURATED FAT: 3.5 grams • CHOLESTEROL: 70 milligrams • SODIUM: 610 milligrams • TOTAL CARBOHYDRATE: 19 grams • FIBER: 1 gram • PROTEIN: 12 grams

Carrot-Raisin
Grain Salad

This salad packs a punch of flavor and texture. Although many people with diabetes believe that raisins are off limits, this dish offers a taste of raisin without being over the top in sugar—the raisins plump up when they're mixed with warm, moist spelt grains. Rugged and earthy, spelt complements the sweetness of raisins nicely.

Serves 6

3 cups low-sodium chicken broth

1 cup spelt berries

1 pound carrots, shredded

½ cup raisins

½ cup walnuts, chopped

2 tablespoons olive oil

1 tablespoon lemon juice

1 teaspoon freshly ground nutmeg

1 teaspoon cinnamon

Salt and freshly ground black pepper

Combine the chicken broth and spelt berries in a medium-size pot, bring to a boil, and cook, covered, until the spelt berries are tender, about 45 minutes. Drain well, discarding any remaining broth.

Toss the warm spelt berries with the remaining ingredients, seasoning to taste with salt and pepper, and mix well. Let stand for about 1 hour at room temperature (this will give the raisins time to plump and the carrots time to soften). Serve at room temperature or refrigerate for up to 1 week.

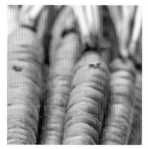

NOTE Spelt is a hardy grain that is similar to common wheat; it is fairly easy to grow, making it an ideal grain to grow organically. It's also high in protein and fiber and has a sweet, nutty flavor—matching the carrots and walnuts nicely in this recipe.

NUTRITION INFORMATION: SERVING SIZE: ½ cup • CALORIES: 260 • CALORIES FROM FAT: 110 • TOTAL FAT: 12 grams • SATURATED FAT: 1.5 grams • CHOLESTEROL: 0 milligrams • SODIUM: 65 milligrams • TOTAL CARBOHYDRATE: 36 grams • FIBER: 6 grams • PROTEIN: 7 grams

Grapefruit Tabbouleh
with Pistachios

Most of the tabboulehs I've tried have been seasoned with lemon and parsley, but this Middle Eastern grain-based salad takes well to experimentation. This recipe is a little sweeter and more filling than traditional versions. The grapefruit offers a sweet, acidic note, and the cucumber and pistachios add a nice crunch.

Serves 8

2 cups chicken broth

1 cup bulgur

3 grapefruits (2 sectioned, 1 zested and juiced)

¼ cup olive oil

1 small red onion, finely chopped

½ English cucumber, finely diced

2 scallions, sliced

½ cup pistachios, chopped

½ teaspoon grated fresh ginger

Salt and freshly ground black pepper

Bring the chicken broth to a boil in a medium-size pot. Add the bulgur, reduce the heat, and simmer, covered, until the bulgur is al dente, about 15 minutes. Drain well, discarding any remaining broth. Chill the bulgur for 2–3 hours.

Finely grate the zest of one grapefruit and then juice it; you should have ½ cup of freshly squeezed juice. Peel the remaining two grapefruits and cut into segments.

Combine the cooled bulgur with the grapefruit segments, juice, and zest, along with the olive oil, onion, cucumber, scallions, pistachios, and ginger. Season to taste with salt and pepper and toss well.

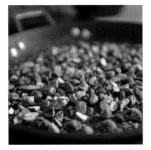

NOTE Oranges get a lot of hype, but grapefruits are also packed with vitamins A and C and may help lower cholesterol. Plus, red and pink grapefruits contain lycopene, a powerful antioxidant that may reduce cancer risk.

NUTRITION INFORMATION: SERVING SIZE: about ½ cup • CALORIES: 180 • CALORIES FROM FAT: 90 • TOTAL FAT: 10 grams • SATURATED FAT: 1.5 grams • CHOLESTEROL: 0 milligrams • SODIUM: 15 milligrams • TOTAL CARBOHYDRATE: 21 grams • FIBER: 4 grams • PROTEIN: 4 grams

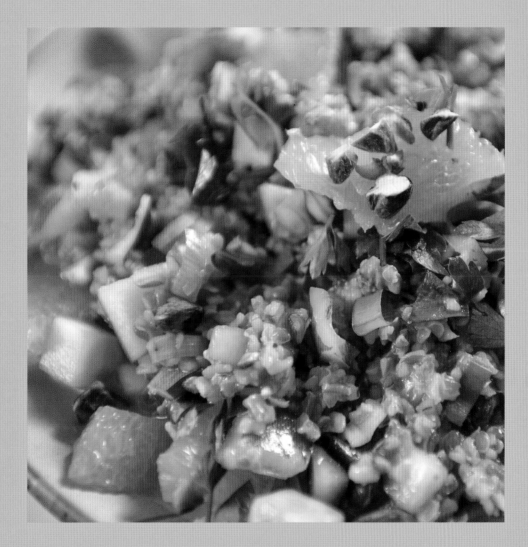

Roasted Fennel, Orange, and Almond
Salad with Tomato Vinaigrette

Fennel usually is considered a fall and winter vegetable, but the first harvest of fennel in the late spring and early summer is especially sweet. In summer, fresh tomatoes make a deliciously light dressing for this salad.

Serves 4

1 sweet onion, cut into ⅛-inch-thick slices

1 bulb fennel, cut into ⅛-inch-thick slices

3 tomatoes, cut into quarters

5 garlic cloves, unpeeled

Leaves from 3 sprigs fresh thyme

Salt and freshly ground black pepper

2 tablespoons olive oil

6 cups arugula

8 radishes, thinly sliced

2 Valencia oranges, peeled and cut into segments

½ cup slivered almonds

Preheat the oven to 425°F. Arrange the onion slices and fennel on one roasting pan and spray lightly with olive oil. Arrange the tomatoes and garlic on another roasting pan. Place the pans in the oven and roast until the onions and fennel are golden and tender, tossing gently halfway through, and the tomatoes have burst, 25–30 minutes. Remove from the oven and transfer to separate plates. Set aside to cool.

Remove the skins from the garlic and place the garlic in a blender along with the roasted tomatoes and thyme leaves; season to taste with salt and pepper. Blend the mixture until smooth and then add the olive oil in a slow drizzle and blend until very smooth.

To assemble the salad, combine the arugula, cooled roasted vegetables, radishes, oranges, and almonds in large bowl. Toss gently with the tomato vinaigrette.

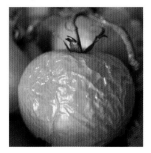

NOTE Fennel has a sweet, light flavor that's been given a bad name by licorice jelly beans. The flavor is much gentler; caramelizing it lightly in the oven mellows the taste further.

NUTRITION INFORMATION: SERVING SIZE: 1 salad • CALORIES: 150 • CALORIES FROM FAT: 80 • TOTAL FAT: 9 grams • SATURATED FAT: 1 gram • CHOLESTEROL: 135 milligrams • SODIUM: 50 milligrams • TOTAL CARBOHYDRATE: 16 grams • FIBER: 5 grams • PROTEIN: 5 grams

Broccoli Sprout Summer Rolls
with Peanut Dipping Sauce

Rice paper is very delicate. You have to soften it in water and place it on a flat, moist surface (I like to use a damp paper towel), and then you place the filling inside and gently wrap the sides. Don't let the filled rolls touch because they'll rip. However, by the third or fourth roll, you'll be churning them out in no time. At that point I encourage you to choose other fillings and try baking or steaming them to create a different texture.

Serves 4

8 Brown Rice Spring Roll Wrappers (or another brand of rice paper wraps, about 10 inches in diameter)

4 baby bok choy, thinly sliced

2 red bell peppers, julienned

1 English cucumber, julienned

4 ounces broccoli sprouts (or alfalfa sprouts)

Dipping sauce

¾ cup peanut butter

6 tablespoons low-sodium soy sauce

3 tablespoons rice vinegar

3 tablespoons water

1 tablespoon sesame oil

Salt and freshly ground black pepper

Fill a medium-size bowl with warm water. Wet a paper towel and squeeze it out so that it is damp. Place it in front of you in the middle of your work surface. Working with one wrapper at a time, dip it in the water and place it on the damp towel. Let the wrapper sit for about 30 seconds to soften. Place a few pieces of bok choy, red pepper, cucumber, and sprouts on the bottom third of the wrapper. Fold the bottom of the wrapper over the filling, fold in the sides, and roll up tightly. Repeat with the remaining wrappers and filling. Arrange the spring rolls on a platter, taking care that they don't touch.

To make the dipping sauce, whisk together the peanut butter, soy sauce, vinegar, water, and sesame oil until smooth. Season to taste with salt and pepper. Serve with the spring rolls.

NOTE Rice paper is a wonderful tool that all diabetic people should use. The wraps are low in calories (about 30 per wrap) and carbs (about 7 grams per wrap), making them a great vessel for vegetables, meats, and seafood. White rice paper wrappers have been around for a while, but brown rice ones are fairly new to the American market. If your local grocer doesn't have them, you can order them online.

NUTRITION INFORMATION: SERVING SIZE: 2 rolls • CALORIES: 350 • CALORIES FROM FAT: 180 • TOTAL FAT: 21 grams • SATURATED FAT: 2.5 grams • CHOLESTEROL: 0 milligrams • SODIUM: 450 milligrams • TOTAL CARBOHYDRATE: 29 grams • FIBER: 6 grams • PROTEIN: 15 grams

Charred Radicchio
with Cashews and Gorgonzola

Radicchio's bitter bite is great in salads and also stands up well to a little heat. This recipe is always a hit at barbecues: the lemon and parsley make it taste fresh and bright, and a hot grill softens the radicchio and gives it a mellow smokiness.

Serves 6

2 lemons

¼ cup olive oil, plus more for spraying

Small handful of fresh parsley leaves, roughly chopped

Salt and freshly ground black pepper

3 heads radicchio, quartered

½ cup crumbled Gorgonzola

½ cup cashew pieces, toasted

Preheat a grill to medium-high. Finely grate the zest of the 2 lemons and then juice them (you should have about ¼ cup of juice). Whisk together ¼ cup olive oil, the lemon zest and juice, and the parsley; season to taste with salt and pepper.

Spray the radicchio with olive oil and arrange it, cut side down, on the grill. Grill until lightly charred, about 30 seconds per cut side. Remove from the heat.

Gently toss the radicchio with the dressing and then sprinkle with the Gorgonzola and cashews.

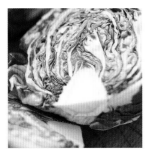

NOTE Radicchio grows best in late summer and early fall, when the temperature is a little cooler and there's a little less light; this helps the plant produce the bright, vibrant purple leaves. Radicchio is high in fiber, vitamin K, and antioxidants, making it a great healthy choice.

NUTRITION INFORMATION: SERVING SIZE: ½ radicchio • CALORIES: 150 • CALORIES FROM FAT: 120 • TOTAL FAT: 13 grams • SATURATED FAT: 4 grams • CHOLESTEROL: 15 milligrams • SODIUM: 180 milligrams • TOTAL CARBOHYDRATE: 5 grams • FIBER: 1 gram • PROTEIN: 4 grams

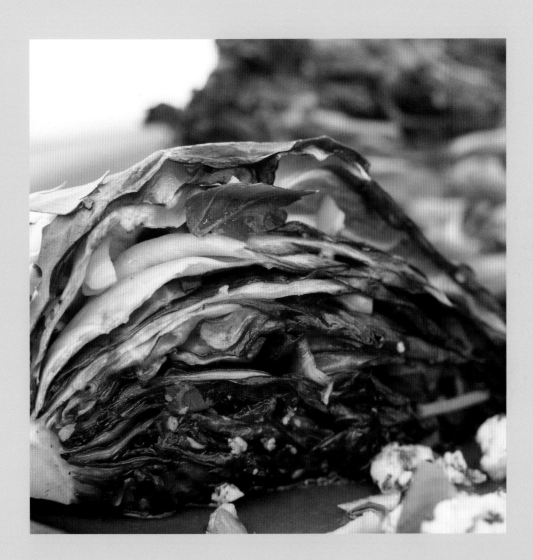

Salmon Carpaccio
on Homemade Bagel Chips

For many people with diabetes, bagels are out of the food rotation. Obviously, because bagels are made from grains, they are high in carbs, but the real problem is portion size: bagels are often double, triple, or even quadruple an appropriate serving size. The solution to a bagel craving? Bagel chips! Baking your own not only is cheaper but results in chips that taste better and have less fat.

Makes 4 bagels or 8 servings*

Whole-wheat everything bagels

- 1 teaspoon active dry yeast
- ½ teaspoon granulated sugar
- ½–⅔ cup plus 1 tablespoon warm water
- 1¾–2 cups whole-wheat flour
- 1¾–2¾ teaspoons kosher salt
- 1 tablespoon olive oil
- 1 egg
- 2 tablespoons dried minced garlic
- 2 tablespoons dried minced onions
- 2 tablespoons sesame seeds
- 2 tablespoons poppy seeds

To make the bagels

In a small bowl, combine the yeast, the sugar, and ½ cup of the warm water. Let stand, without stirring, for 5 minutes.

Meanwhile, combine 1¾ cups flour and ¾ teaspoon salt in a large bowl. Form a well in the middle of the flour. After 5 minutes, stir the yeast and sugar mixture until dissolved and pour it into the flour well and begin mixing. Continue adding a little bit of flour until the dough is firm and moist, or add a little water if it becomes too dry.

Knead the dough on a floured countertop until it's firm and a little stiff, 8–10 minutes. Lightly oil the bowl, and roll the dough around it, oiling all sides. Place a warm, dampened paper towel or clean dish towel over the dough and let it sit in a warm, draft-free place until doubled in size, about 1 hour.

Preheat the oven to 425°F. Bring a large pot of water to a boil. Punch down the dough and divide it into four equal pieces. Roll each into a smooth ball and let sit under a warm, dampened paper towel for about 10 more minutes.

In a small bowl, lightly beat together the egg and 1 tablespoon water to create an egg wash. In a separate bowl, combine the dried garlic, onions, sesame seeds, poppy seeds, and 1–2 teaspoons salt. Set out a large plate and a baking sheet.

Roll each ball of dough into a long log and form it into a circle (creating the bagel), carefully pinching the seam together to seal.

Working in batches, boil the bagels for 2 minutes on each side. Transfer the boiled bagels to the plate and brush with the egg wash. Immediately sprinkle

This recipe makes about four bagels, but the recipe calls for only two, so after the bagels are ready, reserve the remaining two.

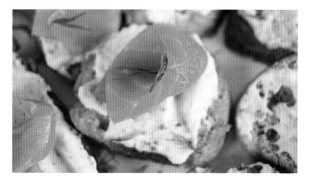

Carpaccio and bagel chips

2 whole-wheat bagels

5 garlic cloves, smashed

2 tablespoons olive oil

8 ounces low-fat cream cheese

¼ English cucumber, grated

Small handful of fresh dill, chopped

1 tablespoon finely grated lemon zest

1 tablespoon lemon juice

Pinch of garlic powder

Salt and freshly ground black pepper

½ pound sushi-grade salmon, cut into 24 (¼-inch-thick) slices

the "everything" mixture over the egg wash. Flip the bagels onto the baking sheet, brush the other side with egg wash, and sprinkle with the everything mixture. Repeat with each bagel until they're all "everything"-ed. Bake, flipping halfway through, until browned on both sides, about 20 minutes.

To make the bagel chips

Preheat oven to 300°F. Heat the garlic cloves and olive oil in a very small pan over low heat until fragrant, 5–6 minutes. Remove from the heat and let cool. Discard the garlic and pour the olive oil into a sprayer. Slice the two bagels crosswise so that you have small rounds, about ¼-inch thick. Lightly spray the bagel pieces with garlic oil and bake, flipping once, until lightly browned, 5–6 minutes.

Combine the cream cheese, cucumber, dill, lemon zest and juice, and garlic powder in a bowl. Season to taste with salt and pepper and mix well. Spread 1 teaspoon of cream cheese dip on each bagel slice and top with a slice of fresh salmon. Serve immediately.

NOTE Although the most popular nutrition benefit may be the high content of omega-3 fatty acids (which improve cardiovascular health, mood, cognition, eyesight, and joints), 4 ounces of salmon also has more than 100 percent of the daily recommended amount of vitamins B_{12} and D.

NUTRITION INFORMATION: SERVING SIZE: ½ bagel (about 6 pieces) • CALORIES: 270 • CALORIES FROM FAT: 110 • TOTAL FAT: 12 grams • SATURATED FAT: 3 grams • CHOLESTEROL: 30 milligrams • SODIUM: 340 milligrams • TOTAL CARBOHYDRATE: 27 grams • FIBER: 3 grams • PROTEIN: 17 grams

Spicy Avocado
Gazpacho

This simple recipe adds a dynamic twist to traditional cold gazpacho. It also makes a great base for an avocado Bloody Mary! Just blend it until completely smooth and feel free to up the spice.

Serves 4

2 ripe avocados, flesh removed from the skin, ¼ diced and reserved

2 garlic cloves

Handful of fresh cilantro leaves

Juice of 1 lime (2–3 tablespoons)

4 cups canned low-sodium diced tomatoes (about one 28-ounce can)

2 red bell peppers, diced

1 cucumber, diced

½ red onion, diced

2 tablespoons grated horseradish

2 tablespoons red wine vinegar

2–3 teaspoons sriracha hot sauce

2 teaspoons Worcestershire sauce

Salt and freshly ground black pepper

Pit and peel the avocados. Dice one-quarter of the avocados and set aside. Put the remaining avocados in a blender or food processor along with the garlic, cilantro, and lime juice. Pulse until the avocados are smooth, adding ½ cup of the diced tomatoes at a time.

Combine the bell peppers, cucumber, red onion, the remaining diced tomatoes, and the remaining avocado in a large bowl. Add the horseradish, red wine vinegar, hot sauce, and Worcestershire sauce, along with the avocado-tomato puree, and mix well. Season to taste with salt and pepper. Serve chilled.

NOTE Some recent research has shown that adding avocados to salads and vegetable dishes improves the body's absorption of nutrients in tomatoes (such as lycopene and beta-carotene). Add healthy fats to salads or soups to maximize the health benefits—just be wary of portion size, because fats add a lot of calories to meals.

NUTRITION INFORMATION: SERVING SIZE: 1½ cups • CALORIES: 260 • CALORIES FROM FAT: 140 • TOTAL FAT: 15 grams • SATURATED FAT: 2 grams • CHOLESTEROL: 0 milligrams • SODIUM: 70 milligrams • TOTAL CARBOHYDRATE: 30 grams • FIBER: 11 grams • PROTEIN: 5 grams

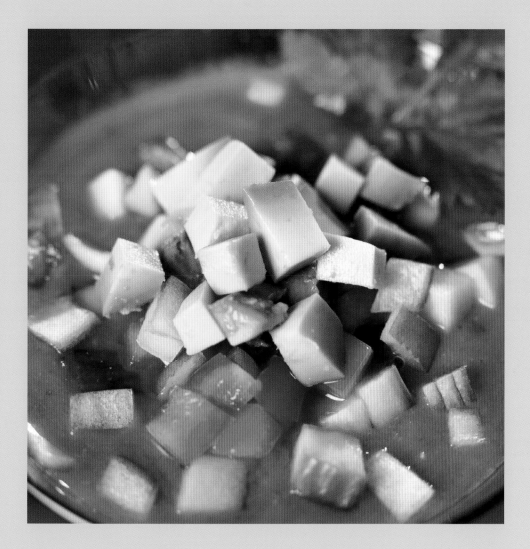

Jalapeño Cornbread Panzanella

For someone with diabetes, one of the easiest ways to enjoy bread is to mix it with vegetables. Here a flavorful cornbread tossed with fresh vegetables, herbs, and a lime-cilantro dressing makes a great appetizer while keeping carbohydrates in check.

Serves 12

Cornbread
- ½ cup buttermilk
- 1½ tablespoons butter, melted
- 2 tablespoons olive oil, divided
- 1 egg
- ½ cup yellow cornmeal
- ¼ cup whole-wheat flour
- ¼ cup all-purpose flour
- 1½ tablespoons sugar
- 1¾ teaspoons baking powder
- ½ teaspoon ground cumin
- ¼ teaspoon baking soda
- ¼ teaspoon paprika
- ¼ teaspoon salt
- 1 jalapeño, seeded and diced
- 1 sweet onion, sliced
- 12 red and yellow cherry tomatoes, halved
- 1 avocado, pitted, peeled, and diced

Preheat the oven to 400°F. Spray an 8 × 8–inch baking dish with vegetable oil.

Mix together the buttermilk, butter, 1 tablespoon olive oil, and egg in a small bowl. Combine the cornmeal, flours, sugar, baking powder, cumin, baking soda, paprika, and salt in a large bowl. Add the wet ingredients to the cornmeal mixture and stir until combined. Fold the jalapeño into the batter and pour into the baking pan. Bake until a toothpick inserted in the center of the bread comes out clean, about 20 minutes. Set aside to cool.

Reduce the oven temperature to 350°F. Cut the cooled cornbread into 1-inch cubes and arrange in a single layer on a baking sheet. Bake the cornbread cubes until golden brown and toasty, about 15 minutes. Set aside to cool.

Meanwhile, heat the remaining 1 tablespoon olive oil in a medium-size saucepan over medium heat. Add the onion and cook, stirring occasionally, until caramelized, about 30 minutes.

To make the dressing

Whisk together the lime juice, olive oil, and cilantro in a small bowl. Season to taste with salt and pepper.

To serve, toss the toasted cornbread with the cherry tomatoes, avocado, and caramelized onions and dressing. Serve immediately.

Dressing

¼ cup freshly squeezed lime juice (from about 5 limes)

2 tablespoons olive oil

Handful of fresh cilantro leaves, finely chopped

Salt and freshly ground black pepper

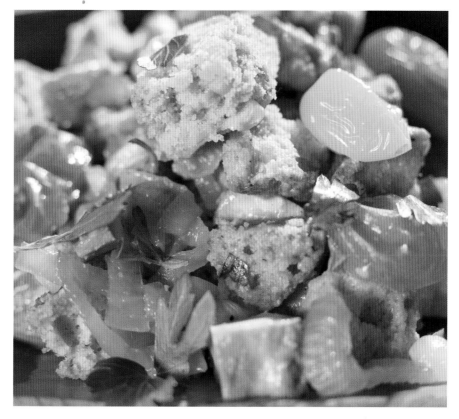

NOTE Cornmeal is a whole grain. It's simply corn that has been dried and milled to a meal (or more finely to a flour). Thus, this recipe is almost 100 percent whole grain. The white, all-purpose flour is a little lighter and improves the texture, but you can substitute whole-wheat flour for the white flour. Using blue cornmeal instead of yellow will give your cornbread an even better nutritional profile.

NUTRITION INFORMATION: SERVING SIZE: ¾ cup • CALORIES: 250 • CALORIES FROM FAT: 120 • TOTAL FAT: 14 grams • SATURATED FAT: 3.5 grams • CHOLESTEROL: 70 milligrams • SODIUM: 320 milligrams • TOTAL CARBOHYDRATE: 27 grams • FIBER: 6 grams • PROTEIN: 6 grams

Watermelon and Tomato
Salad

The first thing that attracted me to combining these fruits was color. Using red, yellow, orange, green, and pink tomatoes combined with red, orange, and yellow watermelon sets the stage for an interesting and unique salad. I love to play with colors when serving this—most people, upon hearing "watermelon and tomato" think red—so try not adding any red or pink. With these two sweet ingredients, cheese and vinegar balance the flavor profile. If you want some added creaminess, try adding avocado.

Serves 4

Dressing
¾ cup balsamic vinegar

Salad
8 sliced watermelon rounds, cut into ½-inch rounds, the same diameter as the tomato slices

4 medium yellow or orange tomatoes, sliced crosswise into ½-inch-thick pieces

4 ounces feta cheese

2 tablespoons thinly sliced fresh mint leaves

1 tablespoon thinly sliced fresh basil leaves

Salt and freshly ground black pepper

In a small saucepan over low heat, reduce the balsamic vinegar by about one-third (about 7 minutes). Using a small cookie cutter, create ½-inch-high rounds of watermelon, tomato, and feta cheese. Pack rounds into one later on a serving platter or plate. Drizzle with reduced balsamic and sprinkle with basil and mint. Salt and pepper to taste.

NOTE Watermelons have far-reaching nutritional benefits, including improving circulation and heart health and reducing the risk of cancer. Because they are 90 percent water, watermelons are also low in calories. Note that yellow watermelons are often sweeter than their red counterparts.

NUTRITION INFORMATION: SERVING SIZE: 1½ cup stack • CALORIES: 220 • CALORIES FROM FAT: 120
• TOTAL FAT: 13 grams • SATURATED FAT: 5 grams • CHOLESTEROL: 25 milligrams • SODIUM: 370 milligrams
• TOTAL CARBOHYDRATE: 19 grams • FIBER: 2 grams • PROTEIN: 7 grams

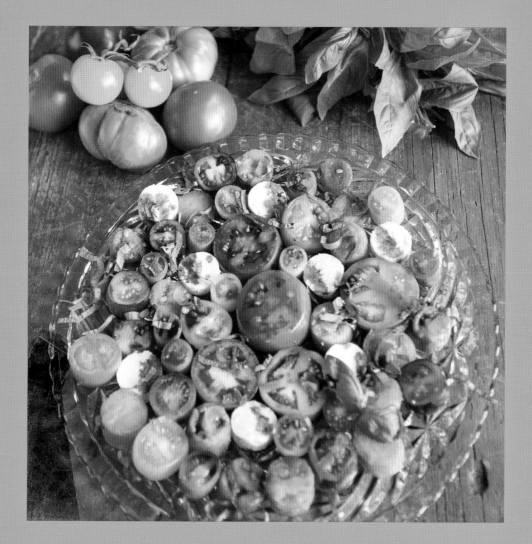

Aleppo-Mustard
Chicken Salad

Chicken salad, which frequently is made with a mayonnaise base, is often high in fat and weak in flavor. Mixing nonfat yogurt with bold, flavorful seasoning instead of mayo creates a healthier and more interesting flavor. Aleppo pepper is only moderate in heat and has a slight smoky sweetness, adding a complex burst of flavor and color.

Serves 4

6 ounces nonfat Greek yogurt

¼ cup buttermilk

2 tablespoons whole-grain mustard

2 tablespoons chopped fresh parsley leaves

1½ teaspoons Aleppo pepper

¼ teaspoon celery salt

1 tablespoon olive oil

Salt and freshly ground black pepper

2 boneless, skinless chicken breasts

6 cups chopped romaine

4 celery stalks, sliced

8 grape tomatoes, quartered

12 olives, pitted and halved

Put the yogurt, buttermilk, mustard, parsley, Aleppo pepper, and celery salt in a bowl and mix until combined. Set aside.

Heat the olive oil over medium heat in a large pan. Season the chicken all over with salt and pepper, add to pan, cover, and cook until the internal temperature (taken with a meat thermometer) reads 165°F, 4–6 minutes per side. Remove from the heat and, when the chicken is cool enough to handle (at least 5 minutes), cut it into cubes. Stir the chicken into the dressing.

Divide the lettuce between four plates. Top each plate with ½ cup of the dressed chicken mixture. Divide the celery, tomatoes, and olives evenly among the plates and serve immediately.

NOTE: Cooking boneless, skinless chicken doesn't often result in the most flavorful dish, but it makes a great base for bolder flavors. The goal for the chicken here is to make sure it stays juicy, which you can do by covering the pan to lock in moisture and making sure to use a meat thermometer. The debate is whether you should let chicken rest after cooking, but for this recipe, you have to let it rest until the chicken is cool enough to handle (just in case, wait at least 5 minutes).

NUTRITION INFORMATION: SERVING SIZE: 1 salad • CALORIES: 180 • CALORIES FROM FAT: 70 • TOTAL FAT: 8 grams • SATURATED FAT: 1 gram • CHOLESTEROL: 35 grams • SODIUM: 610 grams • TOTAL CARBOHYDRATE: 8 grams • FIBER: 1 gram • PROTEIN: 18 grams

5 Easy and Healthy Snacks

1. **Crunchy chickpeas**—Crunchy chickpeas are a great way to have a crunchy, protein-based snack. Check out the recipe on page 88 (with Greek-Style Fish Tacos).

2. **Flavored popcorn**—Air-popped popcorn is easy, low in calories and carbohydrates, and packed with fiber. And you don't need to add butter to make it delicious! Try popping about ½ cup kernels in 2 tablespoons oil over medium heat, covered, shaking occasionally until most of the popping subsides. Then add one of the following combinations: parmesan cheese and finely chopped fresh rosemary, everything bagel seasoning (see page 16 for Salmon Carpaccio and Bagel Chips), chili powder with lime juice, or a little cinnamon-sugar for a sweet treat.

3. **Frozen grapes**—These are best in the summer but still great in the winter. They're super sweet without any added sugar. Remove grapes from stem, rise, and pat dry. Spread in a single layer on a baking sheet and freeze.

4. **Spiced nuts**—Regular nuts can be boring, especially if you want to stay away from all that salt; spiced nuts are a great substitute. Whisk 3 egg whites with 1 teaspoon salt and ¼ teaspoon each of 2–3 favorite spices (like cumin, cayenne, cinnamon, nutmeg, or cloves). Mix the egg white mixture with 4 cups of any type of nut or seed (or a variety of them). Bake nuts in a single layer on a baking sheet at 325°F for about 25 minutes, or until dry.

5. **Roasted edamame**—Roast thawed, shelled edamame drizzled with olive oil and seasoned with salt in a 425°F oven for about 15 minutes (turning 2–3 times). Toss with 1 tablespoon each white and black sesame seeds and roast for about 5 more minutes, or until golden.

Roasted Tomatillo and
Corn Soup

Served hot or cold, this soup screams summer. When tomatillos and corn are in peak season, this soup is sweeter than many desserts. You could even reduce it to about one-third the volume and use it as a dip.

Serves 8

15–20 tomatillos, husks removed and washed

2 tablespoons olive oil

1 large onion, chopped

2–3 cloves garlic, chopped

1 medium jalapeño pepper, chopped

3–4 cups chicken or vegetable stock

4 ears of fresh corn

1 teaspoon ground cumin

Salt and freshly ground black pepper

Fresh cilantro for garnish

Preheat the broiler and lightly spray a roasting pan with olive oil. Place the tomatillos in the pan and broil until charred, about 15 minutes. Remove from the broiler and set aside; keep the broiler on.

Heat olive oil in a large pot over medium-high heat. Add the onion and cook, stirring occasionally, until softened, about 5 minutes. Add the garlic and cook 2–3 minutes more and then stir in the jalapeño. Scrape the tomatillos and their juices from the roasting pan into the pot. Add enough stock to cover the tomatillos, cover, and reduce the heat to medium-low. While the soup is heating up, cut the corn kernels from the cobs (you should have 2–3 cups of kernels). Arrange the kernels in an even single layer on the roasting pan and broil until roasted and browned in spots, 8–10 minutes.

Stir the corn and cumin into the soup. Using a hand blender or food processor, blend the soup until very smooth. Season to taste with salt and pepper. Serve the soup hot or chilled, garnished with a sprig of cilantro.

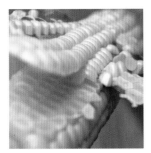

NOTE Tomatillos are very popular in Mexican cuisine and are known as tomate verde ("green tomato"). They have an inedible husk around the outside that turns brown and splits when the tomatillo is mature. Tomatillos are more tart than tomatoes but turn sweeter as they're cooked. They make great sauces, salsas, and soups.

NUTRITION INFORMATION: SERVING SIZE: 1 cup • CALORIES: 130 • CALORIES FROM FAT: 50 • TOTAL FAT: 6 grams • SATURATED FAT: 1 gram • CHOLESTEROL: 0 grams • SODIUM: 50 milligrams • TOTAL CARBOHYDRATE: 18 grams • FIBER: 3 grams • PROTEIN: 4 grams

Black Bean and
Sweet Potato Soup

This soup is one of my favorite wintertime dishes; it's wonderfully filling. Despite the high sugar content of corn, using dried corn for a little crunch is a lot healthier than adding tortilla chips.

Serves 6 (Makes about 8 cups)

1 tablespoon olive oil

1 medium-size yellow onion, chopped

3 stalks celery, chopped

2 large carrots, chopped

3 garlic cloves, minced

Salt and freshly ground black pepper

2 cups dried black beans, soaked overnight

4 cups low-sodium chicken broth

6 tablespoons tomato paste

2 tablespoons chopped chipotle with adobo

1 teaspoon paprika

1 teaspoon ground cumin

½ cup frozen corn, thawed

8 ounces sweet potatoes, diced

Handful of fresh cilantro leaves, roughly chopped

Heat the olive oil in a large pot over medium heat. Add the onion, celery, carrots, garlic, and a pinch of salt and cook, stirring occasionally, until the onions are translucent, 5–6 minutes. Add the black beans, chicken broth, tomato paste, chipotle, paprika, and cumin. Cook, covered, until the black beans are a little underdone, about 1½ hours.

Preheat the oven to 350°F. Pat the corn dry with paper towels and arrange on a small baking sheet. Bake until dry and crunchy, 10–15 minutes. Run under the broiler for an extra 5 minutes if needed.

When the black beans are almost done, remove the lid and add the sweet potatoes. Cook, uncovered, for another 10–15 minutes, until the sweet potatoes are tender and the black beans are al dente (firm but not undercooked). Remove from the heat and puree about half the soup in a blender or with an immersion blender (if you prefer, you can leave the beans whole). Season to taste with salt and pepper.

Ladle the soup into bowls and garnish with the dried corn and chopped cilantro.

NOTE Sweet potatoes that are boiled or steamed have been shown to retain more of their nutritional benefits than sweet potatoes that are roasted. Sweet potatoes are high in beta-carotene (like other deep orange vegetables) but may have their own unique type of antioxidant called sporamin, which may help protect against cancer.

NUTRITION INFORMATION: SERVING SIZE: 1¼ cups • CALORIES: 180 • CALORIES FROM FAT: 30 • TOTAL FAT: 3 grams • SATURATED FAT: 0 grams • CHOLESTEROL: 0 grams • SODIUM: 350 milligrams • TOTAL CARBOHYDRATE: 29 grams • FIBER: 8 grams • PROTEIN: 9 grams

Creamy
Shrimp Bisque

This impressive recipe has zero cream. Though you lose some of a bisque's traditional creaminess, you gain a deep, rich seafood flavor.

Serves 6

1 tablespoon olive oil

1 small yellow onion, chopped

2 carrots, chopped

2 celery stalks, chopped

3 cloves garlic, chopped

1 tablespoon all-purpose flour

2 tablespoons tomato paste

3 cups seafood stock

3 sprigs fresh thyme

2 bay leaves

1 teaspoon smoked paprika

¼ teaspoon cayenne

1 pound deveined, shelled shrimp

1 cup skim milk

6 ounces 2 percent Greek yogurt

Salt and freshly ground black pepper

Heat the oil in a medium-size pot over medium heat. Add the onion, carrots, celery, and garlic and cook, stirring occasionally, until the mixture begins to soften, 2–3 minutes. Add the flour and cook, stirring constantly, for 1 minute. Add the tomato paste, seafood stock, thyme, bay leaves, paprika, and cayenne and bring to a boil. Reduce the heat and simmer for 25 minutes. Add the shrimp and simmer until cooked through, about 5 minutes. Add the milk and yogurt and season with salt and pepper to taste. Discard the thyme sprigs and bay leaves and, using a stick blender or a food processor, puree the soup until very smooth.

NOTE Seafood (or fish) stock is a great alternative to chicken broth. It is nutritionally comparable and naturally complements any fish dish. The downside is that it is very difficult to get low-sodium seafood stock; I'm sure it will come down the pipeline eventually, but right now it's not widely available. Instead, you could make your own low-sodium stock. To do so, save (and freeze) the heads of fish, bones, and other parts (the shells of shrimp). When you have 1 pound of fish parts, (the bones and heads of about 2 medium fish), defrost and cook with 1 cup of white wine, 7 cups of water, 1 chopped yellow onion, 1 bay leaf, 2 sprigs of thyme, 2 minced garlic cloves, 2 chopped carrots, 2 ribs celery, and a pinch of salt. Place all ingredients in a stockpot and bring to a boil. Then simmer, uncovered, until the stock reduces by half and reaches the desired flavor (about 1 hour). Strain thorough a seive, pressing the juices out of the fish parts. Repeat through cheesecloth if necessary.

NUTRITION INFORMATION: SERVING SIZE: 1½ cups • CALORIES: 140 • CALORIES FROM FAT: 30 • TOTAL FAT: 3.5 grams • SATURATED FAT: 0 grams • CHOLESTEROL: 95 milligrams • SODIUM: 970 milligrams • TOTAL CARBOHYDRATE: 12 grams • FIBER: 2 grams • PROTEIN: 16 grams

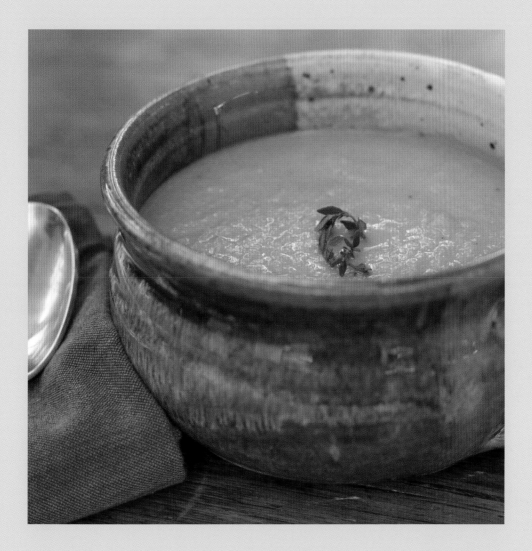

Buffalo
Chicken Cigars

Buffalo chicken wings are a guilty pleasure of mine, but because of the fat content, I eat them only once in a while. I wanted to create a healthier version that capitalizes on their satisfying flavors without capturing the fat. Rosemary, though not traditional, adds a layer of sophistication and dimension without obscuring the essence of a juicy wing with creamy blue cheese. I suggest making a limited number of these because they will go fast.

Serves 10

1 pound ground chicken

¼ cup crumbled blue cheese

¼ cup buffalo sauce

1 tablespoon chopped fresh rosemary

Freshly ground black pepper

10 wonton wrappers

1 egg, lightly beaten with 1 tablespoon water

Spray olive oil

Preheat the oven to 400°F. Working by hand, mix together the chicken, blue cheese (break up the chunks as you work), buffalo sauce, and rosemary. Season with black pepper.

Set 1 wonton wrapper on a work surface, with a corner pointed at you. Place about ¼ cup of the chicken mixture on the corner of the wrapper closest to you. Fold the bottom of the wonton wrapper over the filling and then roll it up, folding the left and right ends in as you go to enclose the filling. Brush the top corner of the wrapper with the egg wash and finish rolling it to seal. Place on a baking sheet and repeat with the remaining chicken mixture and wonton wrappers. Lightly spray the wraps with olive oil before baking

Bake, turning halfway through, until golden, about 20 minutes. Serve warm.

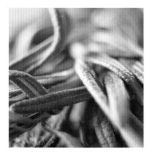

NOTE How much better are these cigars than wings *really*? Well, let's say a serving of wings from your local fast-food eatery or pub is about five wings. Those five wings contain about four times the calories, five times the fat, and four times the sodium of one cigar in this recipe. And unlike the cigar recipe, the calculation for pub wings doesn't include the calories of fat in the typical side of blue cheese dressing.

NUTRITION INFORMATION PER ROLL: SERVING SIZE: 1 • CALORIES: 150 • CALORIES FROM FAT: 50 • TOTAL FAT: 6 grams • SATURATED FAT: 2 grams • CHOLESTEROL: 55 milligrams • SODIUM: 410 milligrams • TOTAL CARBOHYDRATE: 12 grams • FIBER: 0 grams • PROTEIN: 13 grams

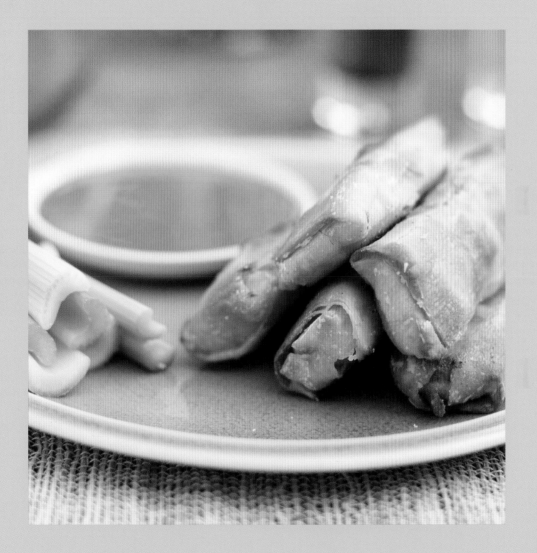

Sunchoke
Chicken Soup

Avgolemono, a Greek chicken soup flavored with lemon, traditionally contains white rice, which isn't so diabetic-friendly. Sunchokes, a starchy root vegetable, are a delicious and healthy alternative. Also known as Jerusalem artichokes, sunchokes are native to North America and were discovered on Cape Cod in the seventeenth century. Knobby, homely looking, and in my opinion underutilized, sunchokes are actually the root of a type of sunflower and have a sweet, nutty flavor.

Serves 6

2 tablespoons olive oil

2 small onions, chopped

8 cups chicken broth

3 celery stalks, chopped

2 carrots, chopped

2½ cups sliced sunchokes

1 leek, chopped

4 cloves garlic, chopped

2 boneless, skinless chicken breasts

2 sprigs fresh rosemary

2 sprigs fresh oregano

2 bay leaves

3 tablespoons cornstarch

½ cup cold water

2 eggs

Finely grated zest and juice of 5–6 lemons

Salt and freshly ground black pepper

4 tablespoons chopped chives

Heat the olive oil in a pot over medium heat and add the onions. Cook, stirring occasionally, until golden, 5–8 minutes. Add the broth, celery, carrots, sunchokes, leek, garlic, and chicken breasts. Make a bouquet garni by placing the rosemary, oregano, and bay leaves on a square of cheesecloth, gathering up the ends and tying it securely. Add the bundle to the broth, cover, and poach the chicken until cooked through, about 15 minutes.

Remove the chicken and herb bundle and set aside. Remove the pot from the heat and, using an immersion blender or food processor, blend the vegetables and broth until smooth. Return the soup to the pot along with the herb bundle, reduce the heat to low, and simmer until reduced by about a third, about 20 minutes.

Meanwhile, cut the chicken into cubes. Combine the cornstarch and cold water in a small bowl and whisk until smooth. In a large bowl, whisk together the eggs and lemon juice.

Stir the cornstarch slurry into the simmering soup, along with the cubed chicken. Whisking constantly, slowly add 2 cups of the hot soup to the egg-lemon mixture. Once it is incorporated, add the mixture back to the soup pot and stir well. Season to taste with salt and pepper. Ladle the soup into bowls and sprinkle with the chives and reserved lemon zest.

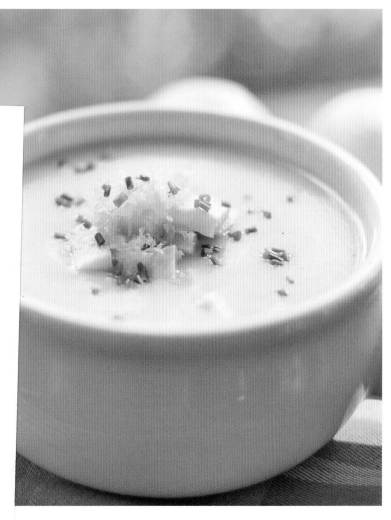

...ORMATION: SERVING SIZE: about 2 cups • **CALORIES:** 170 • **CALORIES FROM FAT:** 50 • **TOTAL ...ATURATED FAT:** 1 gram • **CHOLESTEROL:** 65 milligrams • **SODIUM:** 160 milligrams • **TOTAL ...0 grams • FIBER:** 2 grams • **PROTEIN:** 12 grams

Orange-Ginger
Tuna Ceviche

As the tuna marinates in a bright, citrusy dressing, it develops a sweet, gingery flavor. For an extra kick, sprinkle the tuna with a little chili pepper or add a bit of sriracha sauce to the marinade. As an alternative to tuna (which some believe is too fatty to make good ceviche, though I obviously disagree), choose a whitefish such as grouper or flounder.

Serves 4

5 navel oranges

4–5 limes

2 scallions, finely chopped

1 (1-inch) piece fresh ginger, peeled and grated

2 tablespoons chopped fresh cilantro leaves

2 tablespoons olive oil

Salt and freshly ground black pepper

8 ounces sushi-grade tuna, cut into ⅛-inch slices (about 16 pieces)

2 blood oranges

Finely grate the zest of two of the navel oranges and reserve, then juice them (you should have 2 cups of juice; juice the third orange, if needed). Set the remaining two oranges aside for the salad.

Juice enough of the limes to yield ⅔ cup juice. Whisk together the orange juice, lime juice, scallions, grated ginger, cilantro, and olive oil in a bowl. Season to taste with salt and pepper. Add the tuna to the dressing and refrigerate for 20 minutes.

Meanwhile, peel and slice the blood oranges and reserved navel oranges into thin rounds. Stack a slice of blood orange over a slice of navel orange and top with a slice of tuna. Continue with the remaining orange slices and tuna. Garnish each stack with a drizzle of dressing and a sprinkle of the reserved orange zest.

NOTE Ceviche is a traditional Central and South American dish made by marinating raw fish in citrus juice, and it works with a range of seafood. If scallops or calamari look good at the market on the day you're shopping, they'll work well in this recipe, too.

NUTRITION INFORMATION: SERVING SIZE: 4 rounds • CALORIES: 130 • CALORIES FROM FAT: 25 • TOTAL FAT: 3 grams • SATURATED FAT: 0.5 gram • CHOLESTEROL: 20 milligrams • SODIUM: 20 milligrams • TOTAL CARBOHYDRATE: 13 grams • FIBER: 2 grams • PROTEIN: 14 grams

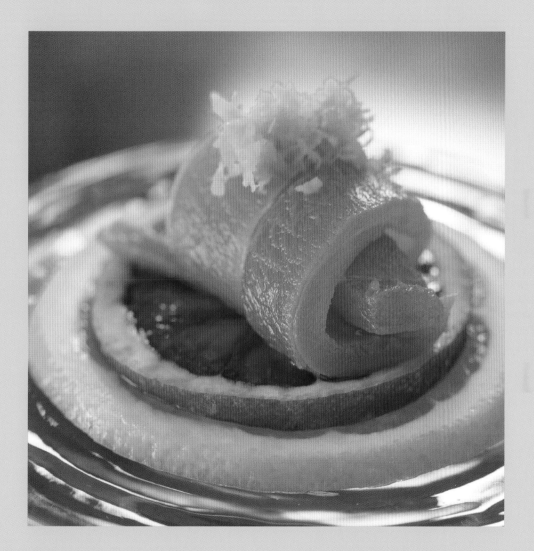

Raw Kale Salad
with Buttermilk Parmesan Dressing

Dinosaur kale (also known as lacinato) is a unique variety—the dark green leaves are stiff and bumpy. It's similar to a hearty lettuce, making it ideal to be eaten raw. Plus, the longer you let the leaves sit in the dressing, the softer the leaves become.

Serves 4

½ cup buttermilk

½ cup grated Parmesan cheese, divided

4 tablespoons red wine vinegar

2 tablespoons olive oil

1 shallot, finely chopped

1 clove garlic, halved

Salt and freshly ground black pepper

8 cups chopped dinosaur kale

4 eggs

2 beets, red or golden, peeled

Whisk together the buttermilk, ¼ cup Parmesan cheese, vinegar, olive oil, shallot, and garlic; season to taste with salt and pepper. Pour the dressing over the kale and toss well to coat. Refrigerate for 10 minutes and then toss again.

Meanwhile, bring a medium-size pot of water to a boil. Place the eggs in the water, reduce the heat, and simmer for 2 minutes. Remove from the heat, cover, and let the eggs sit for 10 minutes. Drain the eggs and let them sit under cold running water until cool. Peel and gently slice each egg, keeping them together.

Using a mandoline, a food processor, or a sharp knife, thinly slice the beets.

Remove the kale from refrigerator and toss again, ensuring that all leaves are coated and are beginning to soften.

To assemble, divide the dressed kale between four plates and top with the sliced raw beets and hard-boiled eggs. Sprinkle the remaining ¼ cup Parmesan cheese over the salads and serve.

NOTE Buttermilk has not received enough attention in recent years. Because it is the result of churning cream for butter (all the fat remains in the butter), buttermilk is naturally low in fat but has a rich flavor. It softens gluten in baking (which makes it great for cakes, in which you don't need a lot of gluten) and helps make salad dressings a little thicker without adding a lot of calories.

NUTRITION INFORMATION: SERVING SIZE: 2 cups kale, 1 egg, ½ beet • CALORIES: 290 • CALORIES FROM FAT: 150 • TOTAL FAT: 17 grams • SATURATED FAT: 5 grams • CHOLESTEROL: 200 milligrams • SODIUM: 390 milligrams • TOTAL CARBOHYDRATE: 21 grams • FIBER: 4 grams • PROTEIN: 17 grams

5 Superfoods for Health

1. **Edamame**—These green beans are high in fiber, with complex carbohydrates, protein, omega-3 fats, and antioxidants. Fresh edamame benefit from a light steam or roast (in their pods), whereas frozen edamame are available shelled and can be used to make hummus or to top salads.

2. **Fresh sardines**—This fish is high in omega-3 fatty acids and protein. Sardines have a short season, but they are fairly inexpensive when they're fresh (Pacific Northwest: July through September; Atlantic, New England: October and November). Fresh sardines are delicious and easy to make; try sautéing the whole fish with oil, or grilling or baking it with lemons and herbs. The canned version gets a bad rap for its scent, but when fresh sardines are unavailable (e.g., out of season), canned sardines can be great broiled.

3. **Chia seeds**—High in omega-3 fats and fiber, chia seeds are very easy to eat! Sprinkle them over salads, add them to oatmeal, or add them to pureed fruit to make a custard-like treat (see page 172 for the Coconut Chia Seed and Lemon Pudding).

4. **Berries**—High in many vitamins, flavonoids, or other antioxidants, berries are versatile and convenient. You can rise and eat them fresh in season (with yogurt and cardamom) or use frozen berries to make smoothies.

5. **Beets**—Yes, you read that correctly! Despite the fact that beets are higher in carbohydrate than some other vegetables, they contain an antioxidant that may help decrease some of the complications of long-term, uncontrolled blood sugar (such as effects to the eyes or nerves). Try beets raw, grated over a salad, or roasted whole. Or pickle them (see How to Make Quick Pickles in 5 Easy Steps on page 39).

Pickled Pear
and Cauliflower Salad

Pickling is not my forte, but this is a recipe with which you really can't go wrong. The pickled pear adds layers of unexpected flavor to the salad and is a good reminder that fruit can be used in many different ways. I chose ginger, cloves, and rosemary for the brine because of their strong, complementary flavors. Reserve the extra vinegar—it can be strained and bottled, making a great homemade gift.

Serves 4

Pickled pears

- 2 cups white vinegar
- 1 cup water
- 1 tablespoon granulated sugar
- 1 tablespoon kosher salt
- 2 sprigs fresh rosemary
- 1 (2-inch) piece of ginger, peeled
- 5 dried cloves
- 2 Bosc pears, cored and cut into ¹⁄₁₆-inch-thick slices

Salad

- ⅓ cup pear vinegar
- 2 tablespoons olive oil
- 1½ teaspoons garlic powder
- Freshly ground black pepper
- 3 cups chopped cauliflower florets
- 1 head green leaf lettuce, roughly chopped
- 4–5 scallions, thinly sliced

Prepare the pears at least 1 day ahead. Bring the vinegar, water, sugar, salt, 1 sprig rosemary, ginger, and cloves to a boil. Reduce the heat to low and simmer for about 5 minutes. Remove from the heat. While the brine simmers, place the pears and remaining 1 sprig rosemary into a clean jar or container with a tight-fitting lid (if you are using mason jars, you might have to cut the pears in half or bend them to fit inside, but they will soften as they pickle and be easier to remove). Pour the hot pickling liquid over the pears and let the liquid cool to room temperature, about 30–60 minutes. Cover the pears and chill for at least 24 hours before using; pears can be made up to 1 week ahead.

To make the salad, strain the pickled pears, reserving the pear vinegar. Whisk together ⅓ cup pear vinegar, the olive oil, and the garlic powder in a small bowl; season to taste with black pepper. Put the cauliflower, lettuce, scallions, and drained pears in a large bowl. Add the dressing and toss gently to combine.

NOTE Pickling is a technique I encourage everyone to try. It's a great way to preserve seasonal fruits or vegetables and creates opportunities to try different flavor combinations (like this recipe's ginger, rosemary, and cloves). Since these pears are not treated with heat, they do not lose any nutrients in the pickling process.

NUTRITION INFORMATION: SERVING SIZE: about 1½ cups salad mixture, ½ pear • CALORIES: 160 • CALORIES FROM FAT: 60 • TOTAL FAT: 7 grams • SATURATED FAT: 1 gram • CHOLESTEROL: 0 milligrams • SODIUM: 55 milligrams • TOTAL CARBOHYDRATE: 23 grams • FIBER: 6 grams • PROTEIN: 4 grams

How to Make Quick Pickles in 5 Easy Steps

1. Choose the vegetable you want to pickle and prepare them. Things that work well are cabbage, beets, cucumbers, or carrots. If you want something more exotic, try okra, green beans, corn, lemons, watermelon rind, or pineapple. Almost any vegetable will work.

      Preparation means washing and chopping into whatever shape you prefer. For some vegetables, like beets, carrots, or okra, blanch the veggies first (briefly cook them in boiling water).

2. Fill pint- or quart-size mason jars with vegetables or fruit. If you don't have mason jars, you can use any heatproof plastic or tempered glass (such as Pyrex) with lids.

3. Choose spices or aromatics. I try to limit the number of herbs, spices, or flavors to three or four. Some ideas for combinations include cinnamon, cloves, and peppercorns (use with grapes or watermelon rind), fennel, garlic and orange (use with cucumbers or just fennel alone), lemon, mustard, and thyme (use with asparagus), or dill, horseradish, and garlic (use with cucumbers or okra). Add these to the jars or containers.

4. Make the pickling liquid (called brine). Some pickling brines are sour, some are sweet, and some are spicy—it depends on what you're pickling. For a good briny base, use equal parts (3 cups each) water and distilled white vinegar, at least 1½ tablespoons salt (use more salt for a saltier pickle, up to 2–3 tablespoons for 6 cups of liquid), and sugar (use 2 tablespoons for a sour or up to 1½ cups for a sweet brine, or any amount in between).

5. Bring your chosen ingredients to a boil and stir until the sugar and salt are dissolved. Carefully pour over vegetables, fruits, herbs, spices, or aromatics into jars. Leave about ½ inch of space at the top of the jar, covering the vegetables or fruit. Place lids on jars and refrigerate for at least 24 hours and up to one month.

Collard-Wrapped Amaranth
with Vodka Sauce

I was about 17 when I started experimenting with cooking, and penne à la vodka was the first recipe I mastered. When I first tried to make it, I asked my mom to take me to the liquor store to buy vodka. She replied, "I think we have some in the liquor cabinet," to which I responded, "We have a liquor cabinet?" Nothing tasted better to me than my first cooking success, despite my parents' 20-year-old vodka. In future iterations, I made it healthier. Here I wanted to cut out the pasta altogether—amaranth is a great substitute! With collard greens as a vessel, the sweet and creamy goodness of the sauce always takes me back to one of the nicer moments of being a teenager.

Serves 5

10 collard leaves

1¼ cups low-sodium chicken broth

½ cup amaranth

1 tablespoon olive oil

3 shallots, finely minced

3 cloves garlic, finely minced

½ cup vodka

1 (14-ounce) can low-sodium crushed tomatoes

1 tablespoon finely chopped fresh oregano leaves

1 tablespoon finely chopped fresh basil leaves

¼ cup light cream

Pinch of crushed red pepper, optional

Salt and freshly ground black pepper

Bring a large pot of water to a boil. Prepare a large bowl filled with ice and cold water. Add the collard leaves to the boiling water, pushing down on them with a spoon to submerge them, and blanch for 2 minutes. Using tongs, transfer the leaves directly to the cold water bath. When the leaves have cooled, remove and pat dry with paper towels.

Bring the chicken broth to a boil in a medium-size saucepan and add the amaranth. Cover and cook until tender, about 20 minutes. Remove from the heat.

In another medium-size saucepan, heat the oil over medium heat. Add the shallot and cook, stirring occasionally, until softened, about 3 minutes. Add the garlic and cook 2 minutes more. Add the vodka and carefully ignite the alcohol with a lighter or match; let the alcohol burn off. When the flame extinguishes itself, add the crusted tomatoes. Bring the sauce to a boil and then add the oregano and basil and continue to cook until the sauce has reduced by a quarter. Reduce the heat to low and add the cream and crushed red pepper, if using. Season to taste with salt and pepper. Simmer the sauce for 2–3 more minutes and then remove from the heat.

To assemble, combine about ¾ of the sauce with the amaranth and mix well. Spoon about ¼ cup amaranth-sauce mixture onto the lower third of a

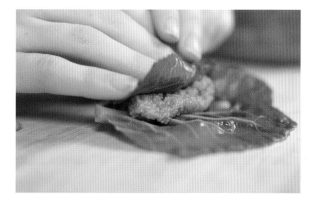

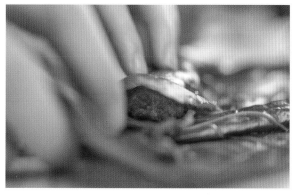

NOTE Amaranth is a grain that's just starting to come on the scene. It can be popped like corn or cooked in water or another liquid to make a porridge-like cereal. Amaranth is higher in protein than any other grain and is an excellent source of calcium and iron.

collard leaf. Roll the mixture into the leaf, tucking in the leaf's sides as you go (as if you were making a burrito with a tortilla). Slice each whole wrap on a bias. Repeat with the remaining leaves, using less amaranth-sauce mixture for the smaller leaves. Spoon the remaining one-quarter of the sauce into a serving dish for dipping.

NUTRITION INFORMATION: SERVING SIZE: 2 wraps • CALORIES: 220 • CALORIES FROM FAT: 80 • TOTAL FAT: 9 grams • SATURATED FAT: 3.5 grams • CHOLESTEROL: 15 milligrams • SODIUM: 400 milligrams • TOTAL CARBOHYDRATE: 27 grams • FIBER: 6 grams • PROTEIN: 7 grams

Herbed Polenta
with Gorgonzola and Mushrooms

Polenta holds up nicely to bold flavors such as rosemary and blue cheese. In this recipe, the lightly seasoned woodsy mushrooms and savory Gorgonzola balance the textures and flavors in the dish. If you want a larger portion, add a few handfuls of spinach and a squeeze of lemon.

Serves 4

1 tablespoon olive oil

8 ounces mushrooms, sliced

1 cup low-sodium chicken or vegetable broth

¾ cup cornmeal

2 cloves garlic, minced

2 teaspoons chopped fresh rosemary

1 tablespoon butter

Salt and freshly ground black pepper

½ cup crumbled Gorgonzola

Heat the olive oil in a medium-size pan over medium-high heat. Add the mushrooms and cook, stirring occasionally, until browned on both sides, about 8–10 minutes. Remove from the heat.

Bring the broth to a boil in a medium-size pot over medium-low heat. Add the cornmeal, garlic, and rosemary and cook, stirring constantly, until the mixture thickens, about 10 minutes. Remove from the heat, stir in the butter, and season with salt and pepper.

To serve, top ½ cup polenta with mushrooms and Gorgonzola.

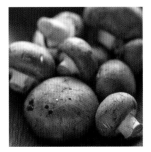

NOTE Rosemary adds a bold, piney fragrance and flavor to dishes. Though usually consumed in small amounts, it is high in iron and vitamins A and C and has health benefits such as stimulating the immune system, increasing circulation and blood flow to the brain, and reducing inflammation. Historically it is also known for improving memory,

NUTRITION INFORMATION: SERVING SIZE: ½ cup prepared polenta • CALORIES: 210 • CALORIES FROM FAT: 110 • TOTAL FAT: 12 grams • SATURATED FAT: 6 grams • CHOLESTEROL: 25 milligrams • SODIUM: 460 milligrams • TOTAL CARBOHYDRATE: 22 grams • FIBER: 2 grams • PROTEIN: 7 grams

5 Facts about Alcohol and Diabetes

Alcohol can be a scary word for those with type 2 diabetes, but it doesn't have to be! With these five facts, you can consume alcohol responsibly.

1. General health recommendations state that men should have no more than two drinks per day and women should have no more than one drink per day. One drink equals 12 ounces of beer, 5 ounces of wine, or 1½ ounces of a distilled spirit (not liqueurs).

2. Despite popular belief, alcohol does not break down into sugar, but there are very small amounts of sugar in alcoholic beverages. For instance, wine is made by fermenting grapes, and grapes have sugar. Fermenting sugar results in alcohol, and any unfermented sugar remains in the wine.

3. Wine, beer, and distilled liquors have a glycemic index of zero, which means the very small amount of sugar left after the fermentation process of wine and beer has no impact on your blood sugar or insulin production.

4. Distilled spirits (such as vodka or gin) have no carbohydrates, but the mixers used with them are often very high in sugar. So if you choose a gin and tonic, the only carbohydrates are from the tonic water (in 1 cup of tonic, about 21 grams). In restaurants that use mixes for drinks such as margaritas, the carbohydrate content can be as high as 100 grams or higher! So the carbohydrate content of mixed drinks can add up quickly.

5. Don't drink on an empty stomach. Alcohol may actually cause your blood sugar to decrease; because consuming alcohol causes a release of insulin, your blood sugar goes down.

Shaved Brussels Sprouts
with a Fried Egg and Spiced Pine Nut Crumble

This recipe tastes rich without being high in fat or calories. I'm normally a multiple-herb-and-spice kind of gal, but this needs no extra attention. The egg yolk adds just enough body and complements the hearty greens. If you want to incorporate even more protein, add some extra egg whites, which will pair nicely with the spiced pine nut crumble.

Serves 4

½ cup pine nuts

1½ teaspoons paprika

1 tablespoon olive oil, plus more for spraying

1 pound Brussels sprouts, trimmed and very thinly sliced using a knife, mandoline, or food processor

Salt and freshly ground black pepper

½ cup grated Parmesan

Pinch of crushed red pepper

4 eggs

Pulse the pine nuts and paprika together in a food processor until combined and roughly chopped, 5–10 seconds.

Heat the olive oil in a medium-size skillet over medium-high heat. Add the Brussels sprouts, season to taste with salt and pepper, and cook, stirring occasionally, until the sprouts are bright green and golden-brown in spots, about 5 minutes. Remove from the heat and stir in the Parmesan and crushed red pepper; set aside.

Lightly spray another large skillet with olive oil and heat over medium heat. Crack the eggs into the skillet and fry, without turning, until the whites are set but the yolks are still runny. Remove from the heat.

To serve, divide the Brussels sprouts among four plates and top each plate with a fried egg and a sprinkle of the nut crumble.

NOTE Many herbs and spices have nutritional and health benefits, but often, to get the benefits, you have to consume a lot. Paprika, however, is not one of those spices. It comes in a variety of types (e.g., sweet, spicy, smoked), all of which contain vitamins A, B_6, and E, plus iron and capsaicin. Capsaicin is the ingredient in chili peppers that can help with pain relief (it's often an ingredient in over-the-counter topical skin creams).

NUTRITION INFORMATION: SERVING SIZE: ½ cup Brussels sprouts • CALORIES: 320 • CALORIES FROM FAT: 220 • TOTAL FAT: 24 grams • SATURATED FAT: 5 grams • CHOLESTEROL: 200 milligrams • SODIUM: 310 milligrams • TOTAL CARBOHYDRATE: 11 grams • FIBER: 5 grams • PROTEIN: 16 grams

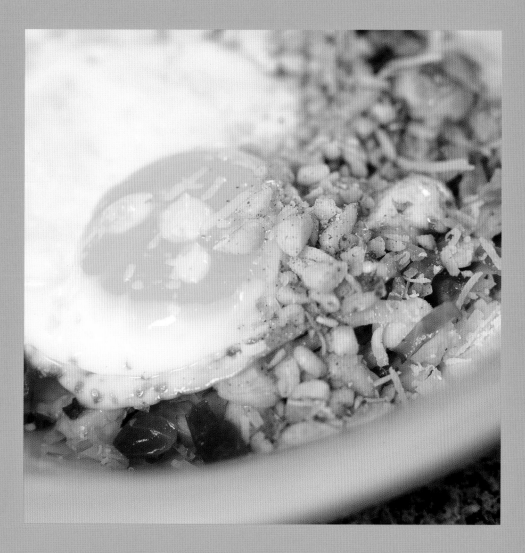

Main Dishes

In the United States, main dishes are notorious high-carbohydrate meals. This does not have to be the case. Instead, let creativity be the key—you want an entrée to be filling but not pose a risk to your health by causing a blood sugar spike. And though creating main dishes with meat or fish is a great way to keep the carbohydrate content low, a plant-based whole-food lifestyle is also important.

Consequently, this section consists mainly of "combination" dishes—meat or fish and vegetables or grains—that help achieve a balance of plant- and meat-based meals. Recipes such as Mustard-Crusted Salmon over Buttermilk Creamed Kale, Smoked Gouda and Broccoli Lasagnettes, and Roasted Poblano Peppers with BBQ Pulled Chicken are hearty and filling and raise the bar for "diabetic" recipes.

(continued on next page)

Mango-Turkey Burger

After I stopped eating red meat at 13 years old (a lifestyle choice I upheld for nearly 18 years), turkey burgers became a summer staple. Often, however, the burger would be dry or tasteless. Then, one year, at my family's annual Father's Day cookout, my aunt prepared turkey burgers with a few tablespoons of mango salsa (a recipe she read about somewhere), and I knew she was onto something. Though any type of salsa would add great flavor, fresh mangoes and jalapeños provide a great sweet and spicy balance while keeping the burger moist.

Serves 4

¾ cup finely diced mango

¼ red onion, finely diced

1 jalapeño, finely diced

Juice of 1 lime

Salt and freshly ground black pepper

1½ pounds lean ground turkey

4 whole-wheat sandwich thins

½ avocado, pitted, peeled, and thinly sliced

Combine the mango, red onion, jalapeño, and lime juice in a small bowl and season to taste with salt and pepper. Let sit for at least 1 hour or refrigerate as long as overnight.

Preheat a grill to medium-high. In a large bowl, mix together the ground turkey and the mango salsa. Gently shape into four 6-ounce patties.

Brush the grill with a towel soaked in olive oil to prevent the meat from sticking. Grill the burgers until cooked through, about 3–4 minutes per side. Remove from the grill and arrange in the sandwich thins. Top each burger with a few slices of avocado.

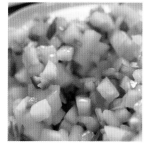

NOTE Mangoes can be grown outdoors only in the southernmost regions of the East Coast and in southern California, but mango trees can survive indoors during the winter in cooler climates. If mangoes aren't locally available in your area and you don't want to buy frozen, use peaches instead.

NUTRITION INFORMATION: SERVING SIZE: 1 burger, plus sandwich thin • CALORIES: 320 • CALORIES FROM FAT: 60 • TOTAL FAT: 7 grams • SATURATED FAT: 0.5 gram • CHOLESTEROL: 50 milligrams • SODIUM: 250 milligrams • TOTAL CARBOHYDRATE: 29 grams • FIBER: 5 grams • PROTEIN: 37 grams

Red Pepper and Artichoke Ravioli
with Walnut Tarragon Pesto

Rarely do I meet ravioli I don't like. These are great for spring: the vegetable-to-cheese ratio makes them light but filling, and the pesto, made with tarragon and walnuts rather than basil and pine nuts, is very interesting.

Serves 6 • Makes: about 30 ravioli

6 tablespoons olive oil, divided

¼ cup finely chopped Vidalia onion

1 clove garlic, minced

¾ cup chopped walnuts

Leaves from 3 sprigs fresh tarragon

Salt and freshly ground black pepper

2 red peppers, cored, seeded, and finely diced

½ cup finely chopped frozen artichoke hearts, thawed

½ cup part-skim ricotta

1 tablespoon fresh thyme

30 wonton wrappers

Heat 3 tablespoons of the olive oil in a medium-size pan over medium heat. Add the onion and reduce the heat to medium-low. Cook, stirring occasionally, until golden and caramelized, about 20 minutes. Add the garlic and cook until fragrant, 2–3 minutes. Remove from the heat.

Meanwhile, pulse the walnuts, tarragon, and the remaining 3 tablespoons of olive oil in a food processor until smooth. Season to taste with salt and pepper and pulse to combine. Set aside.

Stir together the caramelized onion, red peppers, artichoke hearts, ricotta, and thyme in a medium-size bowl. Season to taste with salt and pepper.

Fill a small bowl with warm water. Place one wonton wrapper on a clean work surface and spoon about 1 teaspoon of the filling on the center of the wrapper. Brush the edges of the wrapper with water and fold over to form a triangle, sealing the edges. Repeat with the remaining wontons and filling.

Bring a large pot of water to a boil. Gently add the ravioli and cook until tender, about 3 minutes. Remove the ravioli with a slotted spoon and immediately toss with the pesto (this will prevent them from sticking together).

NOTE Wonton wrappers are a great substitute for pasta dough because they're easy to use, thin, and light, with fewer calories and carbohydrates than regular pasta.

NUTRITION INFORMATION: SERVING SIZE: 5 ravioli • CALORIES: 360 • CALORIES FROM FAT: 190 • TOTAL FAT: 21 grams • SATURATED FAT: 3.5 grams • CHOLESTEROL: 10 milligrams • SODIUM: 290 milligrams • TOTAL CARBOHYDRATE: 35 grams • FIBER: 5 grams • PROTEIN: 10 grams

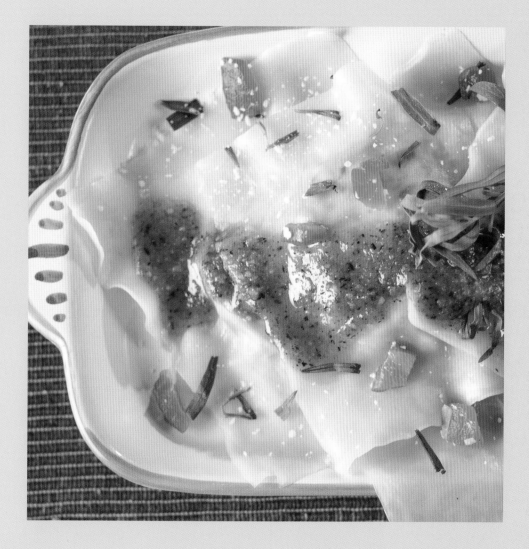

Wild Mushroom Risotto
with Seared Red Snapper and Cilantro Chimichurri

I love the contrast of meaty mushrooms and the fresh taste of cilantro. The red snapper is the perfect bridge between the two flavors.

Serves 4

Handful of fresh cilantro leaves

Juice of 1 lime (about 1½ tablespoons)

2 tablespoons plus 1 teaspoon olive oil

1 teaspoon white vinegar

Salt and freshly ground black pepper

¾ ounce dried porcini mushrooms

1½ cups hot water

4 cups low-sodium chicken broth, or as needed

12 ounces baby bella mushrooms, sliced

½ yellow onion, chopped

2 cloves garlic, minced

¾ cup arborio rice

Olive oil spray

4 (6-ounce) fillets red snapper

To make the chimichurri, put the cilantro, lime juice, 2 tablespoons olive oil, and vinegar in a food processor or blender and pulse to combine; season to taste with salt and black pepper. Set aside.

Cover the dried porcini mushrooms with 1½ cups hot water and set aside to soak. Heat the chicken broth until warm over medium-low heat; keep warm.

Heat the remaining 1 teaspoon olive oil over medium-high heat in a large saucepan. Add the mushrooms and cook, stirring occasionally, until browned, 5–8 minutes. Reduce the heat to medium, add the onion, and cook, stirring occasionally, until softened, 5–6 minutes. Add the garlic and cook 2–3 minutes more. Stir in the rice and about 1 cup of the mushroom soaking liquid (pour carefully to keep any sediment from the mushrooms inside the bowl, not in the risotto, and leaving the porcini mushrooms to continue soaking).

Once the mushroom liquid is absorbed, add 1 cup warm chicken broth to the rice mixture, stirring until the broth is fully absorbed before adding the next bit of broth. Continue adding broth, ½ cup at a time, until the rice is tender and the risotto is creamy. Remove from the heat and cover to keep warm.

Lightly spray a medium-size pan or grill pan with olive oil and heat at medium-high. Season the red snapper with salt and pepper and arrange in the hot pan. Cook the fish until golden and cooked through, 2–3 minutes per side. Remove from pan and add the porcinis; sauté 4–5 minutes or until golden.

To serve, spoon about ½ cup risotto into a warmed bowl and top with a snapper fillet, a few tablespoons of porcinis, and a drizzle of chimichurri.

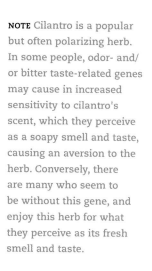

NOTE Cilantro is a popular but often polarizing herb. In some people, odor- and/or bitter taste-related genes may cause in increased sensitivity to cilantro's scent, which they perceive as a soapy smell and taste, causing an aversion to the herb. Conversely, there are many who seem to be without this gene, and enjoy this herb for what they perceive as its fresh smell and taste.

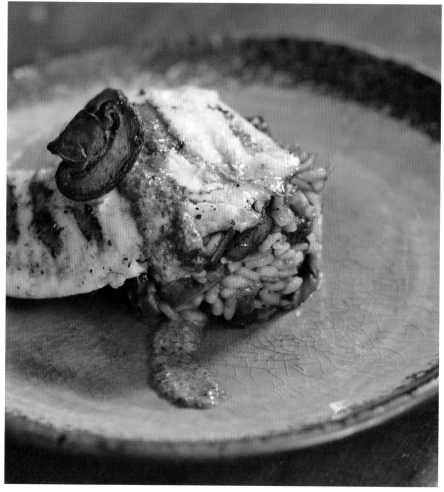

NUTRITION INFORMATION: SERVING SIZE: ⅓ cup risotto, 1 fish fillet • CALORIES: 470 • CALORIES FROM FAT: 100 • TOTAL FAT: 12 grams • SATURATED FAT: 1.5 grams • CHOLESTEROL: 80 milligrams • SODIUM: 520 milligrams • TOTAL CARBOHYDRATE: 37 grams • FIBER: 4 grams • PROTEIN: 53 grams

Spicy Buckwheat
Noodle Soup

As the oppressiveness of winter begins to lighten, so do my meals. As a New Yorker, I still want warming dishes because the spring here isn't always warm, but I don't want heavy meals. This soup is both warming and light. Plus, it provides a great opportunity to use whatever extra vegetables you might have.

Serves 6

8 cups low-sodium chicken broth

8 cups water

3 tablespoons miso

1 teaspoon garlic powder

1 teaspoon Chinese five-spice powder blend

6 eggs

6 ounces buckwheat soba noodles

12 ounces fresh mushroom mix (porcini, shitake, cremini), very thinly sliced

3 heads baby bok choy, chopped

2 carrots, shredded

2 jalapeños, thinly sliced

2 teaspoons sriracha sauce

1 teaspoon grated fresh ginger

6 scallions, sliced

Combine the chicken broth, water, miso, garlic powder, and Chinese spice blend in a large pot and bring to a boil. Boil uncovered, for about 10 minutes.

Meanwhile, bring a medium pot of water to a boil. Reduce the heat to just below a simmer and gently place the eggs in the water. Cook for 6 minutes and then remove from the heat and fill the pot with cold water to cool the eggs.

While the eggs are cooling, add the noodles to the broth and cook until slightly undercooked, about 6 minutes. Add the mushrooms, bok choy, carrots, jalapeño, sriracha sauce, and ginger to the broth. Reduce the heat to low and simmer just until the noodles are tender. Remove from the heat.

Carefully remove the shells from the eggs. Ladle the soup into six bowls, using tongs for the noodles if necessary. Place an egg in each bowl and sprinkle scallions on top. To eat, cut into the egg and stir the yolk into the broth.

NOTE Buckwheat often is used as a cover crop, that is, a crop grown to inhibit the growth of weeds, build nutrient-rich soil, and help control pests. However, it can be made into a porridge using the berry or processed into flour and used to make noodles. Buckwheat is high in protein and both soluble and insoluble fiber (which together help control blood sugar, cholesterol, and keep the digestive tract healthy).

NUTRITION INFORMATION: SERVING SIZE: 2 cups of soup • CALORIES: 240 • CALORIES FROM FAT: 50 • TOTAL FAT: 6 grams • SATURATED FAT: 1.5 grams • CHOLESTEROL: 185 milligrams • SODIUM: 620 milligrams • TOTAL CARBOHYDRATE: 33 grams • FIBER: 4 grams • PROTEIN: 16 grams

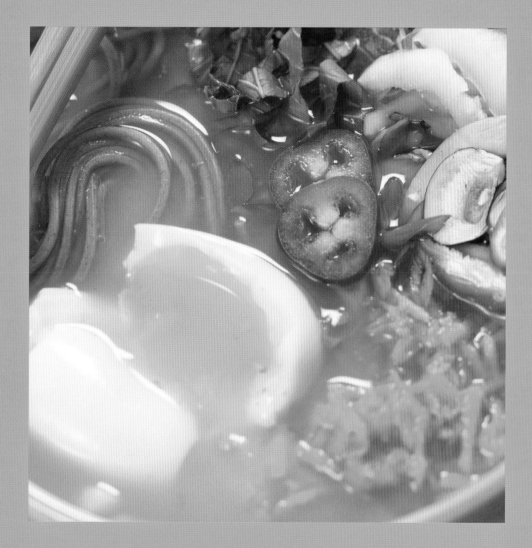

Coconut-Crusted Chicken
in a Curry Broth

Loving Indian flavors doesn't always mean loving Americanized Indian food, so much of which leans heavily on rice and fats such as ghee. But this easy broth is a light—in flavor and in spice intensity—way to enjoy curry.

Serves 6

2 cups whole-wheat panko

1 cup unsweetened coconut flakes

2 teaspoons Madras curry powder, divided

1 teaspoon turmeric, divided

½ teaspoon garlic powder

½ teaspoon garam masala

½ teaspoon paprika

Salt and freshly ground black pepper

1 cup buttermilk

1 (13.5-ounce) can unsweetened coconut milk, divided

6 boneless, skinless chicken breasts

1 tablespoon olive oil

6 shallots, chopped

3 cloves garlic, minced

4 cups low-sodium chicken broth

½ teaspoon ground ginger

¼ teaspoon cumin

6 tablespoons sliced scallions

Preheat the oven to 350°F. Lightly spray a baking sheet or roasting pan with olive oil. Stir together the panko, coconut flakes, 1 teaspoon curry powder, ¾ teaspoon turmeric, garlic powder, garam masala, paprika, and a dash of salt and pepper in a wide bowl. In a separate wide bowl, combine the buttermilk with ⅓ cup of the coconut milk. Dip each chicken breast in the buttermilk mixture, then dredge in the panko mixture and place on the baking sheet. If you have extra panko mixture, feel free to dredge the chicken breasts a second time. Bake until cooked through, 25–30 minutes.

Meanwhile, heat the olive oil in a medium-size saucepan over medium heat. Add the shallots and cook, stirring occasionally, until translucent, about 6 minutes. Add the garlic, stir, and cook for another 2–3 minutes. Add the chicken broth, remaining coconut milk, ginger, cumin, remaining 1 teaspoon curry powder, and remaining ¼ teaspoon turmeric. Salt and pepper to taste. Bring to a simmer and cook until reduced by about half, about 10 minutes.

To serve, ladle ½ cup of broth in a bowl, add a chicken breast, and top with 1 tablespoon scallions.

NOTE Although curry often is thought of as heavy and pungent, when used sparingly, it can be light and subtle. Madras curry powder, one of many types of curry powders from around the globe, was originally a south Indian variety (the Madras region). It is spicy and often is used with meats, poultry, and/or coconut; it can be found in most grocery stores.

NUTRITION INFORMATION: SERVING SIZE: 1 chicken breast and ½ cup broth • CALORIES: 480 • CALORIES FROM FAT: 240 • TOTAL FAT: 26 grams • SATURATED FAT: 21 grams • CHOLESTEROL: 75 milligrams • SODIUM: 270 milligrams • TOTAL CARBOHYDRATE: 29 grams • FIBER: 5 grams • PROTEIN: 35 grams

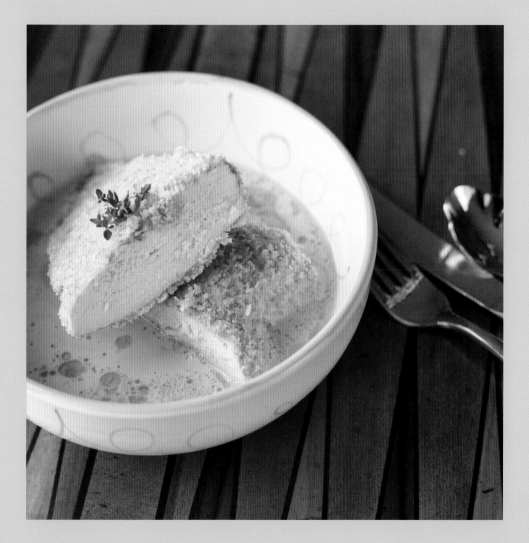

Sautéed Branzino
with a Beluga Lentil and Spinach Ragout

Branzino, also known as Mediterranean sea bass, is one of my favorite varieties of fish. Hands down. Ever. It's light, flaky, and rich in flavor. I first discovered it at a little restaurant in Astoria, Queens, an area known for its large Greek population. On a good day, you'll wait only about 30 minutes for a table during prime dinner hours, but I have happily waited up to an hour and a half. Every time I order the branzino, and every time I think it's the best I've ever had. Although I can't replicate this restaurant's years of experience, I have had a lot of success cooking branzino at home.

Serves 4

3 teaspoons olive oil, divided

1 carrot, chopped

1 small onion, chopped

2 cloves garlic, minced

¾ cup beluga (black) lentils, rinsed and drained

2 tablespoons chopped fresh thyme leaves

1½ cups low-sodium chicken broth

1½ cups shredded spinach

Salt and freshly ground black pepper

4 (6-ounce) branzino fillets

2 tablespoons chopped fresh basil leaves

Heat 2 teaspoons olive oil in a medium-size saucepan over medium heat. Add the carrot and onion and cook, stirring occasionally, until softened, about 5 minutes. Add the garlic and cook 2–3 minutes more. Add the lentils, thyme, and broth; bring to a simmer; and cook, uncovered, for about 15 minutes. Stir in the shredded spinach and cook until the lentils are tender, about 5 minutes. Season to taste with salt and pepper. Keep warm.

Heat the remaining 1 teaspoon oil in a large, heavy pan over medium heat. Season the branzino fillets with salt and pepper and cook them, 2 fillets at a time, until golden brown and cooked through, 2–3 minutes per side.

To serve, spoon some of the lentil mixture on each plate and top with a branzino fillet and fresh basil.

NOTE Mediterranean sea bass is obviously not regional for Americans, but there are fish farms in the United States that are (supposedly) growing branzino sustainably, making it locally available to many people. However, a similar type of fish would be one that is white, lean, and flaky, such as rainbow trout or whiting.

NUTRITION INFORMATION: SERVING SIZE: 1 fillet and ⅓ cup ragout • CALORIES: 330 • CALORIES FROM FAT: 60 • TOTAL FAT: 7 grams • SATURATED FAT: 1 gram • CHOLESTEROL: 55 milligrams • SODIUM: 140 milligrams • TOTAL CARBOHYDRATE: 30 grams • FIBER: 7 grams • PROTEIN: 37 grams

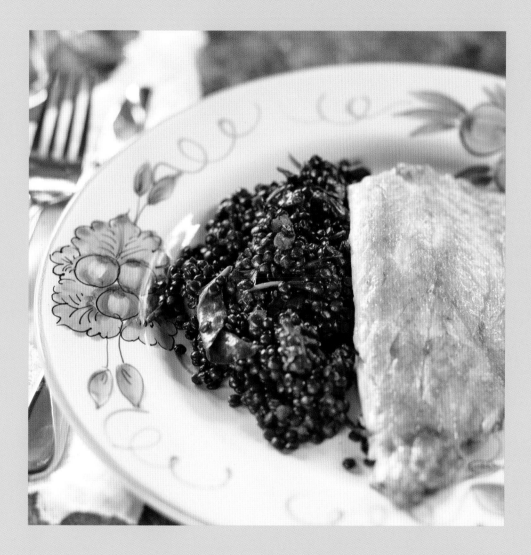

Panko-Crusted Cod
with a Garlic-Lemon Aioli

I didn't like fish as a kid, probably because my exposure was limited to the processed fish sticks offered in the school cafeteria. When I finally had real pieces of fish crusted and baked, I was amazed at the difference. Cod is a great fish to use in this recipe, but you also can choose haddock or pollock.

Serves 4

Cod

- 1 pound fresh cod, rinsed and patted dry
- ½ cup all-purpose flour
  Salt and freshly ground black pepper
- 2 large egg whites, beaten
- 1 cup whole-wheat panko
- 2 tablespoons finely chopped fresh parsley leaves
- 1 tablespoon ground fennel seeds
- 1 teaspoon garlic powder
- ½ teaspoon cayenne

Aioli

- Finely grated zest and juice of 1 lemon
- 1 egg yolk
  Salt and freshly ground black pepper
- 1 large clove garlic, minced
- ½ cup vegetable oil or as needed

Preheat the oven to 375°F. Cut the cod into 24 even pieces. Put the flour in a shallow bowl and season with salt and pepper; mix well. Put the egg whites in another shallow bowl and beat together lightly. In a third shallow bowl, combine the panko, parsley, fennel seeds, garlic powder, and cayenne. Dredge each piece of cod in the flour mixture, dip in the egg whites, and then coat well with the spiced panko. Transfer the cod to a lightly oiled baking sheet. Repeat until all the cod is coated.

Bake the cod until the crust is golden and crisp and the fish is cooked through, about 7 minutes.

Meanwhile, make the aioli. Put the lemon zest, lemon juice, egg yolk, salt, pepper, and garlic in a blender and blend until smooth. Add the oil in a thin stream until the mixture becomes creamy and thick.

Serve the panko-crusted cod with the aioli.

NOTE Cod is high in vitamins and low in fat. The fat that it does have contains a lot of omega-3 fatty acids, which may help improve cardiovascular health, protect against cancer, and help prevent and control high blood pressure. Most cod is a relatively good choice in terms of sustainability and is fairly inexpensive.

NUTRITION INFORMATION: SERVING SIZE: 6 pieces cod, 1 tablespoon aioli • CALORIES: 400 • CALORIES FROM FAT: 170 • TOTAL FAT: 19 grams • SATURATED FAT: 3 grams • CHOLESTEROL: 215 milligrams • SODIUM: 120 milligrams • TOTAL CARBOHYDRATE: 27 grams • FIBER: 2 grams • PROTEIN: 29 grams

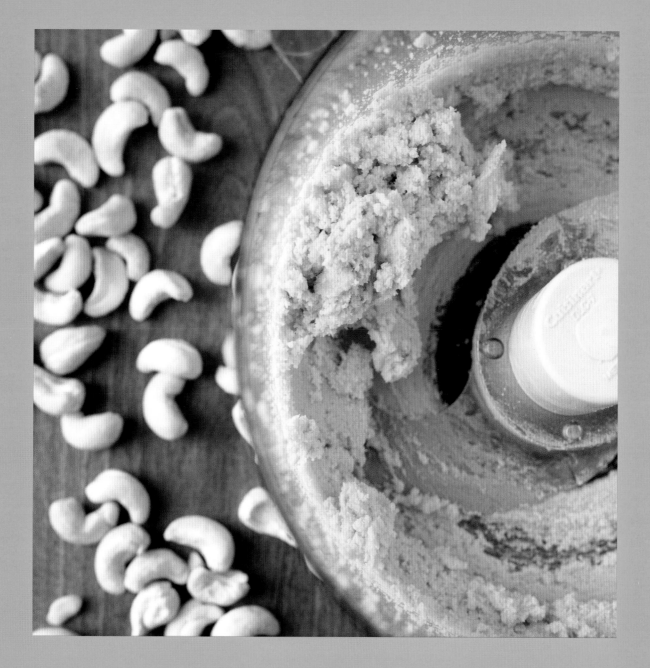

Champagne-Garbanzo Ratatouille

Ratatouille is one of those dishes that I didn't appreciate as a child, but when I started working in farmers' markets, the whole world of eggplant-based ragouts came alive. Champagne is an unusual addition to ratatouille, but I find that using just a little adds great depth of flavor (this is a great opportunity to use some leftover champagne that has lost its effervescence). I prefer dry (brut) champagnes, which are the lowest in sugar. If you have another wine on hand, feel free to use it in this recipe, but remember, the more sweet the wine, the more sugar it has.

Serves 8–10

2 tablespoons olive oil

1 medium onion, chopped

2 cloves garlic, minced

3 large ripe tomatoes, cored and chopped

2 red bell peppers, diced

1 eggplant, diced

3 cups low-sodium chicken broth, divided

6 tablespoons tomato paste

1 bay leaf

1 cup quinoa

2 teaspoons garlic powder

1 (15-ounce) can chickpeas, rinsed and drained

½ cup champagne

1 tablespoon chopped fresh thyme

1 tablespoon chopped fresh rosemary

Salt and freshly ground black pepper

1 cup grated Parmesan

Heat the oil in a large pot over medium heat. Add the onion and cook, stirring occasionally, until slightly softened, 3–4 minutes. Add the garlic and cook until fragrant, 1–2 minutes. Add the tomatoes, red peppers, eggplant, 1 cup chicken broth, tomato paste, and bay leaf. Bring to a simmer, cover, and cook for about 30 minutes.

Meanwhile, bring the remaining 2 cups of chicken broth to a boil in a medium-size saucepan and then add the quinoa and garlic powder. Reduce the heat, cover, and simmer until quinoa is tender, 12–15 minutes. Remove from the heat and drain.

Add the chickpeas, champagne, thyme, and rosemary to the ratatouille. Simmer, uncovered, for about 5 minutes or until it reaches the desired consistency. Season to taste with salt and pepper.

To serve, spoon the quinoa into bowls, top with ratatouille, and sprinkle with Parmesan.

NOTE Champagne is packed with polyphenols, nutrients that you may have heard improve memory and brain power. Moderate consumption of wine (about 1 glass per day for women and 2 glasses for men) also may help protect against memory-related aging, reduce the risk of heart attack (and stroke), and promote longevity. Be careful, though, as those with diabetes should consume alcohol only with food.

NUTRTION INFORMATION: SERVING SIZE: 1 cup • CALORIES: 300 • CALORIES FROM FAT: 90 • TOTAL FAT: 10 grams • SATURATED FAT: 3.5 grams • CHOLESTEROL: 15 milligrams • SODIUM: 480 milligrams • TOTAL CARBOHYDRATE: 34 grams • FIBER: 7 grams • PROTEIN: 14 grams

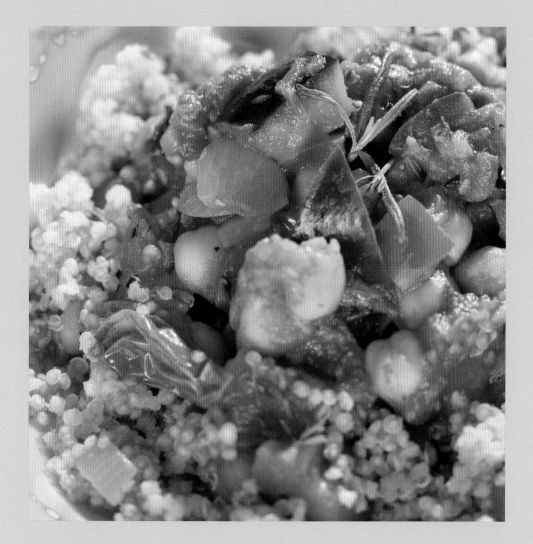

Walnut-Turkey Meatballs
in Pomodoro Sauce

Juicy meatballs without the fat and extra carbs (from a lot of breadcrumbs) are hard to come by. This recipe adds breadcrumbs but creates more flavor by including walnuts, which enhance the flavor and texture without adding saturated fat.

Serves 4

Pomodoro sauce

- 2 tablespoons olive oil
- 1 large sweet onion, finely chopped
- 3 garlic cloves, minced
- 16 plum tomatoes, cored and roughly chopped
- 1 tablespoon dried thyme
- 1 tablespoon dried winter savory
- Salt and freshly ground black pepper

Meatballs

- 1 pound ground turkey
- 2 eggs, beaten
- ½ small onion, minced
- 2 cloves garlic, chopped
- ½ cup whole-wheat panko
- ½ cup grated Parmesan
- ¼ cup walnuts, pulsed in a blender
- 3 tablespoons chopped fresh oregano leaves
- 1½ teaspoons ground cumin

Heat the olive oil in a large pot over medium heat. Add the onion and cook, stirring occasionally, until softened, 4–5 minutes. Add the garlic and cook 2–3 minutes more. Add the chopped tomatoes, thyme, savory, and salt and pepper and cover. Cook, stirring occasionally, until broken down and chunky, 45 minutes to 1 hour.

Meanwhile, put all the meatball ingredients in a large bowl and mix gently with your hands to combine. Scoop up about 2 tablespoons of the mixture, shape into a ball, and arrange on a tray or baking sheet. Repeat with the remaining mixture; you should have about 12 meatballs.

Heat a large pan, sprayed lightly with oil, over medium heat. Working in batches, arrange the meatballs in the pan without crowding and cook, gently rotating them from time to time, until browned on all sides. Ladle some of the tomato sauce into the pan. Remove meatballs and sauce from pan and repeat with the others; it will take two or three batches to complete all the meatballs.

NOTE Portion control is the key to maintaining a healthy weight and can even help people lose weight. It's not always easy to control portions when you're, say, making a large batch of meatballs, which is why using a measuring spoon is important. Two tablespoons equals 1 ounce, and so four meatballs will equal about 4 ounces of meat, an appropriate portion size.

NUTRITION INFORMATION: SERVING SIZE: 4 meatballs • CALORIES: 390 • CALORIES FROM FAT: 160 • TOTAL FAT: 18 grams • SATURATED FAT: 4 grams • CHOLESTEROL: 145 milligrams • SODIUM: 280 milligrams • TOTAL CARBOHYDRATE: 22 grams • FIBER: 5 grams • PROTEIN: 40 grams

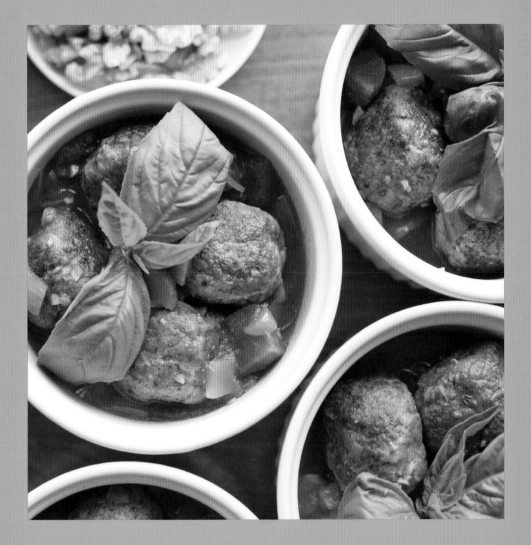

Mustard-Crusted Salmon
over Buttermilk Creamed Kale

Rich salmon and piquant mustard go hand in hand, and this recipe shows off that affinity to great effect. This crust is intensely flavored and bakes up crispy, and so a little goes a long way! If you let the salmon sit out for about 20 minutes before baking, the crust will have time to lose some moisture, ensuring its crunchiness.

Serves 6

Salmon

- 2 pounds salmon
- Salt and freshly ground black pepper
- ½ cup whole-wheat panko
- 2 tablespoons Dijon mustard
- 2 tablespoons whole-grain mustard
- 2 tablespoons white wine
- Handful of fresh parsley leaves, chopped

Buttermilk creamed kale

- 1 tablespoon olive oil
- 1 medium yellow onion, finely chopped
- 2 garlic cloves, minced
- ½ teaspoon paprika
- 2 bunches kale (about 8 cups, chopped)
- 3 cups buttermilk
- 1 cup grated Parmesan

Preheat the oven to 375°F. Rinse the salmon, pat dry, and season with salt and pepper. Place the salmon, skin side down, on a baking sheet.

Stir together the panko, mustard, white wine, and parsley in a small bowl. Spread an even layer of the mustard seasoning over the salmon flesh. Let sit at room temperature for about 20 minutes. Bake the salmon until the internal temperature registers about 145°F on a meat thermometer and the flesh flakes easily with a fork, about 15 minutes.

Meanwhile, heat the olive oil in a medium-size saucepan over medium heat. Add the onion and cook until softened, about 6 minutes. Stir in the garlic and paprika and then add the kale and cook, stirring occasionally, until the kale is bright green, about 6–8 minutes. Drain any excess liquid from the pan and then transfer the kale mixture to a blender or food processor with the buttermilk and Parmesan. Season to taste with salt and pepper and blend until creamy. Return the creamed kale to the pan and bring to a simmer over medium-low heat.

To serve, cut the salmon into six portions and serve with the creamed kale.

NOTE Mustard is a great choice for a condiment: it's low in calories and most mustards don't have added sugar or salt (although there are a few exceptions, like Dijon). There are many types of mustard seeds, which grow in temperate climates such as North America, Europe, and Asia. Mustard is high in antioxidants and phytonutrients, which have a protective effect against cancer. Surprisingly, mustard also has omega-3 fatty acids, making it a great-tasting and great nutritional accompaniment to salmon.

NUTRITION INFORMATION: SERVING SIZE: 5–6 ounces salmon, ½ cup kale • CALORIES: 490 • CALORIES FROM FAT: 210 • TOTAL FAT: 24 grams • SATURATED FAT: 8 grams • CHOLESTEROL: 90 milligrams • SODIUM: 690 milligrams • TOTAL CARBOHYDRATE: 24 grams • FIBER: 3 grams • PROTEIN: 44 grams

Wasabi
Salmon Burger

This burger is the American equivalent of a delicious spicy salmon sushi roll. It takes all the ingredients—the fish, the spice, and the carbohydrate—and the beauty with which these ingredients complement each other to a new, more affordable (and just as healthy) level. Though making these burgers with fresh salmon can get expensive, I'm happy to share this shortcut: this recipe also works with canned salmon, which often has more omega-3s than its fresh counterpart. Also, wild-caught canned salmon is often low in toxins and can be better for the environment (depending on how close you live to where the salmon is caught). Although eating local is preferable, sometimes eating sustainably and affordably wins.

Serves 4

1½ pounds salmon, fresh or canned

½ cup whole-wheat panko

2 teaspoons wasabi paste

2 teaspoons low-sodium soy sauce

1 teaspoon finely grated ginger

4 whole-wheat sandwich thins

1 avocado, pitted, peeled, and thinly sliced

If using fresh salmon, remove and discard the skin. Chop the meat finely with a very sharp knife. Mix the chopped (or canned) salmon with the panko, wasabi, soy sauce, and ginger. Shape the mixture into four patties.

If using a grill, preheat the grill to medium-high and oil the grate lightly before grilling the salmon burgers, about 2–3 minutes per side. If using a pan, spray a large pan with olive oil and place it over medium-high heat. Place the patties in the pan and cook for 2–3 minutes per side.

Serve the burgers on sandwich thins, topped with a few slices of avocado.

NOTE Most wasabi on American shelves is not real wasabi; it is merely horseradish mixed with mustard seed (and dyed green). But you wouldn't know this unless you scrutinized the ingredients on the label. Why would food marketers bother? Well, wasabi is hard to grow, making it extremely expensive, so remember to read the ingredient list before you make a purchase.

NUTRITION INFORMATION: SERVING SIZE: 1 burger • CALORIES: 360 • CALORIES FROM FAT: 160 • TOTAL FAT: 18 grams • SATURATED FAT: 4 grams • CHOLESTEROL: 55 milligrams • SODIUM: 320 milligrams • TOTAL CARBOHYDRATE: 23 grams • FIBER: 5 grams • PROTEIN: 27 grams

Cold Peanut
"Noodles"

My family didn't eat out much when I was growing up, but when we ordered Chinese food, we always got cold spicy noodles. They were my favorite despite being one of the least healthy things on the menu. However, with a couple of nutritional upgrades, cold spicy noodles can be a guilt-free food. Salting the raw vegetables before tossing them with the dressing helps soften them so that their texture is more like cooked pasta.

Serves 4

3 zucchini

1 cucumber

½ cup kosher salt

½ cup freshly ground peanut butter

3 tablespoons low-sodium soy sauce

2 tablespoons sesame oil

2 tablespoons water, or as needed

1 tablespoon rice wine vinegar

1 tablespoon brown sugar

2 teaspoons sriracha sauce

1 head bok choy, shredded

1 bunch scallions, finely chopped

4 tablespoons chopped peanuts

Using a mandoline fitted with the julienne attachment, shred the zucchini and cucumber lengthwise (to get spaghetti-like ribbons). Place the vegetables in a colander in the sink and toss with the kosher salt. Let sit for about 10 minutes to soften, and then drain.

Meanwhile, in a small bowl, whisk together the peanut butter, soy sauce, sesame oil, water, vinegar, brown sugar, and sriracha sauce until smooth, adding a little more water if sauce is too thick.

After 10 minutes, rinse the zucchini and cucumber and drain well. Pat the vegetables dry with paper towels and then transfer them to a large bowl, along with the bok choy and scallions. Pour the dressing over the vegetables and toss well. Garnish with chopped peanuts.

Note: Don't use a processed brand of peanut butter for this recipe. Instead, choose freshly ground peanuts or check the ingredient list on the label, which should list only peanuts (and maybe a little salt) but no added oils or sugar.

NOTE Peanuts are an interesting nutritional conundrum. Because they are often highly processed into butters that include sugar, salt, and oil, most peanut butters are unhealthy. However, peanuts themselves (and peanut butters without added ingredients) are a great source of protein, folate, and vitamin E. They also contain resveratrol, an antioxidant that got a lot of press back in the early 2000s, among other nutrients that make peanuts a great healthy choice.

NUTRITION INFORMATION: SERVING SIZE: 2 cups "noodles" • CALORIES: 420 • CALORIES FROM FAT: 260 • TOTAL FAT: 29 grams • SATURATED FAT: 4 grams • CHOLESTEROL: 0 milligrams • SODIUM: 680 milligrams • TOTAL CARBOHYDRATE: 30 grams • FIBER: 8 grams • PROTEIN: 17 grams

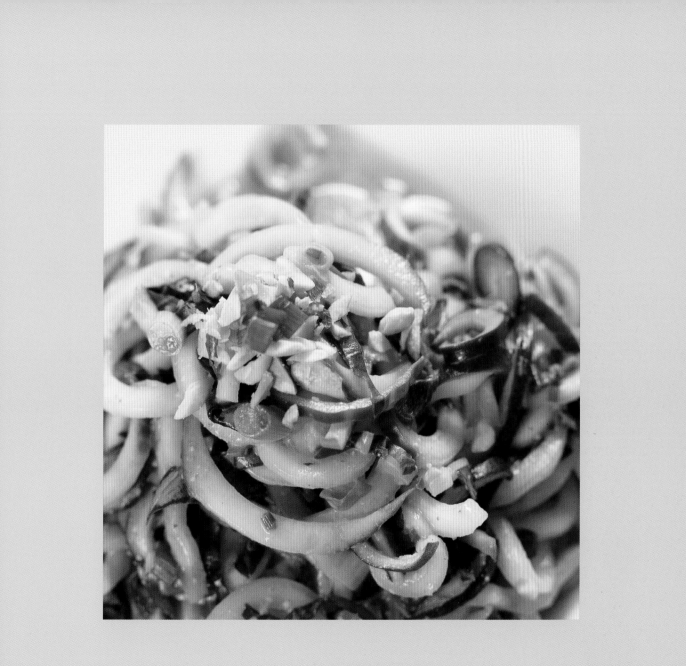

Ginger Soy
Tilapia

Grated ginger, soy, and miso create more of a wet rub than they do a marinade. A little ginger here goes a long way even though the fish is steamed for only a few minutes. The bold flavors of this wet rub respect the delicacy of the fish but give a lot of flavor to what can sometimes be a little too delicate.

Serves 4

2 tablespoons white miso

2 tablespoons low-sodium soy sauce

2-inch piece of ginger, peeled and finely grated

4 (6-ounce) tilapia fillets

1 bunch scallions, roughly chopped

Preheat the oven to 375°F. Stir together the miso, soy sauce, and ginger and gently spread on the tilapia fillets. Cover and refrigerate to marinate for at least 30 minutes.

Set a steamer basket in a wok or a pot, add enough water so that the steamer base sits in the water but the tray sits above it, and bring to a boil. Line the basket with parchment paper to keep the fish from sticking. Place the fish in the basket and scatter the scallions over them. Cover and steam until the fish is opaque and flakes easily, about 6–8 minutes.

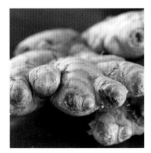

NOTE Tilapia from the United States is a great sustainable choice for fish. Most U.S. tilapia is farmed in a "recirculating system," meaning an indoor facility (pond) covered by greenhouse roofs. Isolating them from wildlife and local water sources ensures an added level of environmental protection, and waste from these facilities is pretty low. Of course, when purchasing fish, you always want to ask your fishmonger where it's from and do research about what the facilities are like at the fishery.

NUTRITION INFORMATION: SERVING SIZE: 1 fillet • CALORIES: 130 • CALORIES FROM FAT: 20 • TOTAL FAT: 2 grams • SATURATED FAT: 0.5 gram • CHOLESTEROL: 55 milligrams • SODIUM: 420 milligrams • TOTAL CARBOHYDRATE: 5 grams • FIBER: 2 grams • PROTEIN: 24 grams

Swordfish Kebabs
with Kiwi, Cherry Tomatoes, and Red Onion

Swordfish is a meaty, juicy fish that is often very expensive. Using it for kebabs lets you enjoy it while saving money. Fruit helps balance the savory marinade and the meatiness of the fish. If kiwis aren't available, try another kind of tropical fruit.

Serves 4

¾ cup nonfat Greek yogurt

Handful of fresh parsley leaves, chopped

½ teaspoon paprika

Salt and freshly ground black pepper

1½ pounds swordfish, cut into 1-inch cubes (yield about 24 pieces)

16 cherry tomatoes

4 kiwis, peeled and quartered

½ red onion, cut into 1-inch squares

Stir together the yogurt, parsley, and paprika in a large bowl; season with salt and pepper. Add the swordfish cubes, mix well until the fish is completely coated, and marinate, covered, in the refrigerator for 1 hour.

Meanwhile, if using wooden skewers, soak them in water for at least 30 minutes.

Preheat a grill to medium-high and lightly oil the grill to keep the skewers from sticking. Thread 3 pieces of swordfish, 2 cherry tomatoes, 2 pieces of kiwi, and 4–6 squares of red onion on each skewer, alternating the pieces of fruit, fish, and vegetables as you like.

Grill the skewers, turning two to three times throughout cooking, until grill marks appear and the fish is cooked through, about 3 minutes per side.

NOTE Swordfish has less cholesterol and nearly 30 percent more protein than an equivalent piece of salmon or lobster and has seven times more healthy fats than tuna. However, because swordfish is high on the food chain, it is high in mercury, so choose swordfish only occasionally. But when you do, you'll know you're making a very healthy choice!

NUTRITION INFORMATION: SERVING SIZE: 2 kebabs • CALORIES: 330 • CALORIES FROM FAT: 110 • TOTAL FAT: 12 grams • SATURATED FAT: 3 grams • CHOLESTEROL: 110 milligrams • SODIUM: 160 milligrams • TOTAL CARBOHYDRATE: 16 grams • FIBER: 3 grams • PROTEIN: 39 grams

Heirloom Tomato and Smashed Olive
Phyllo "Pizza"

Pizza is a treat no matter how you slice it, and a few easy adjustments, such as using fresh tomatoes in place of sauce, can make it healthier. By replacing regular dough (which can be difficult to form into a thin crust pizza) with phyllo dough, you can cut out virtually all the guesswork when it comes to pizza portions. A few sheets of phyllo are all you need to make a delectable thin crust pizza.

Serves 4

½ cup part-skim ricotta cheese

¾ cup grated Parmesan

2 tablespoons chopped fresh oregano leaves

½ teaspoon garlic powder

Salt and freshly ground black pepper

10 sheets phyllo dough, defrosted

2 large ripe tomatoes, preferably a mixture of heirloom varieties, sliced

½ cup yellow cherry tomatoes, sliced

8 Kalamata olives, pitted and roughly chopped or torn

8–10 basil leaves, thinly sliced

Preheat the oven to 400°F. In a small bowl, mix together the ricotta, Parmesan, oregano, and garlic powder; season to taste with salt and pepper. Set aside.

Lay one sheet of phyllo in the center of a nonstick baking sheet. Spray lightly with olive oil and layer another sheet right on top. Repeat with the remaining phyllo sheets. Spread the ricotta mixture evenly over the phyllo, leaving a 1- or 2-inch border on all sides. Arrange the tomatoes over the ricotta mixture, spacing them out fairly evenly. Scatter the olives and sliced basil over the top.

Bake until phyllo edges are lightly brown and crispy and the cheese is melted, 20–25 minutes. Cut using a sharp knife or pizza cutter and serve immediately.

NOTE Like olive oil, olives are high in healthy (monounsaturated) fats and antioxidants and have anti-inflammatory properties. Olives are too bitter to eat off the tree; this is why "virgin" and "extra virgin" oils often taste bitter (they are unrefined) and have the most nutrients. Olives must be cured to be edible; this usually is done with water, brine, salt, or lye.

NUTRITION INFORMATION: SERVING SIZE: 2 slices • CALORIES: 360 • CALORIES FROM FAT: 170 • TOTAL FAT: 19 grams • SATURATED FAT: 8 grams • CHOLESTEROL: 40 milligrams • SODIUM: 860 milligrams • TOTAL CARBOHYDRATE: 33 grams • FIBER: 2 grams • PROTEIN: 16 grams

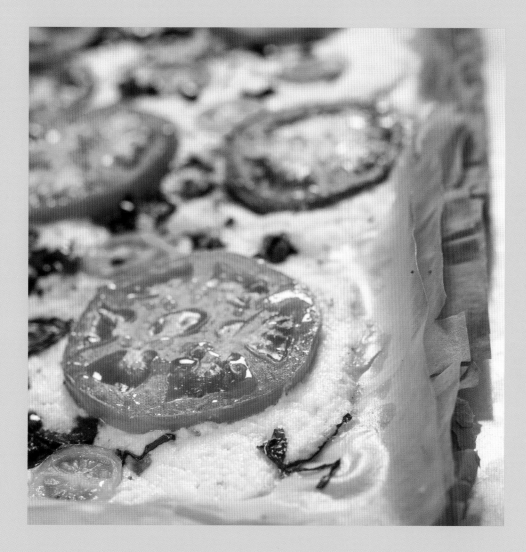

Rainbow Vegetable
Terrine

Roasting vegetables is easy but can be boring. This terrine perks up the old standby with herbs and creamy ricotta. Of course, choosing lots of different colored veggies packs this dish with vitamins and minerals. Feel free to have fun and play with different herbs for this recipe.

Serves 6

4 yellow crookneck squash

4 zucchini

1 eggplant, sliced

¼ cup kosher salt

5–6 large Swiss chard leaves

4 red bell peppers, cored and cut into wide wedges

5 carrots, peeled and thinly sliced lengthwise

4 tablespoons olive oil, divided

Salt and freshly ground black pepper

2 cups part-skim ricotta cheese

3 cloves garlic, minced

2 tablespoons chopped fresh rosemary

2 tablespoons chopped fresh thyme

Cut the yellow squash and zucchini into 5-inch pieces crosswise and then thinly slice lengthwise. Place the eggplant, yellow squash, and zucchini in a colander set in the sink and toss with ¼ cup kosher salt. Let sit while you prepare the rest of the dish.

Preheat the oven to 425°F. Bring a medium-size pot of water to a boil. Fill a bowl with ice and cold water. Add the chard leaves to the boiling water and cook until pliable but still bright green, 2–3 minutes. Transfer to the ice water bath to cool and halt the cooking process. When the leaves are cool, drain them and pat them dry with paper towels.

Place the red pepper and carrots on a baking sheet, drizzle with 2 tablespoon olive oil, and season lightly with salt and pepper. Roast until the skins have browned, about 10 minutes. Transfer the peppers to a plate and set aside.

Meanwhile, line an 8 × 4–inch loaf pan or a similarly sized reusable plastic container with plastic wrap. Arrange overlapping chard leaves along the bottom and up the sides of the pan, letting the leaves hang over the sides of the pan (they will be folded over the top of the completed dish).

Rinse the salted vegetables, drain well, and place on the baking sheet. Drizzle the vegetables with the remaining 2 tablespoons olive oil and season lightly with salt and pepper. (I like to add a little cayenne pepper to the eggplant to give it a little kick and/or add dried oregano to the squash.) Roast the vegetables until lightly browned, about 10 minutes.

NOTE: If I haven't stressed the benefits of "eating the rainbow" enough, this dish is a good plug for it. Eating a variety of colors of fruits and vegetables ensures that you're getting all the vitamins, minerals, and phytonutrients that vegetables have to offer. Phytonutrients often differ by color (e.g., red fruits and vegetables have the phytonutrient lycopene), so be sure to make this dish as colorful as you can!

Stir together the ricotta, garlic, and herbs in a small bowl and season with salt and pepper. Now you're ready to assemble the dish.

I like to follow the order of the colors of the rainbow, so start by adding a layer of red peppers to the bottom of the pan. Layer the carrots over the peppers, pressing down with a flat spatula to even out and pack the layers tightly. After the carrots, use about half the ricotta mixture to create a cheesy layer. Next, repeat with the yellow squash and zucchini, press down, add a layer of cheese, and finally add the eggplant. Press down one last time and tightly fold the leaves over the eggplant layer. Wrap tightly with plastic wrap and refrigerate until firm.

To serve, unmold the terrine, remove the plastic wrap, and cut into 1½-inch-thick slices.

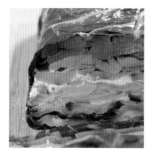

NUTRITION INFORMATION: SERVING SIZE: 1 slice • CALORIES: 330 • CALORIES FROM FAT: 150 • TOTAL FAT: 17 grams • SATURATED FAT: 6 grams • CHOLESTEROL: 25 milligrams • SODIUM: 210 milligrams • TOTAL CARBOHYDRATE: 32 grams • FIBER: 10 grams • PROTEIN: 16 grams

Hazelnut-Crusted Tofu

I think the key to all tofu dishes is not only the flavor but also the texture of the other ingredients in the dish. In the right combinations, tofu can be a meal all on its own. In this case, lemon and hazelnut are not only a natural pairing but also bold enough to give tofu some personality. When tofu is paired with a juicy green such as watercress, the flavors and textures balance one another nicely.

Serves 4

3 lemons, zested to yield at least 1 teaspoon and juiced to yield about ⅓ cup

1 cup skinned hazelnuts

4 sprigs fresh thyme, divided, leaves stripped

½ teaspoon ground cumin

Salt and freshly ground black pepper

2 eggs

2 tablespoons water

3 tablespoons whole-wheat flour

1 pound tofu, cut into 12–14 planks

3 tablespoons olive oil

6 cups chopped watercress

Preheat the oven to 425°F. Finely grate the zest of the lemons to measure 1 teaspoon. Juice the lemon; you should have about ⅓ cup.

Put the hazelnuts, half of the thyme leaves, cumin, and lemon zest in a food processor; season with salt and pepper. Pulse until the mixture is combined and the nuts are fairly well chopped; transfer to a plate.

Lightly beat the eggs and water in a bowl. Sprinkle the flour on a plate. Pat the pieces of tofu with a paper towel and then dredge them in the flour, dip in the egg mixture, and dredge in the hazelnut mixture to coat. Arrange the coated tofu evenly on a baking sheet that has been sprayed lightly with olive oil. Bake, flipping once halfway through, until golden and crisp, about 20 minutes.

Mix the lemon juice, olive oil, and remaining thyme together and toss with the watercress. Serve tofu over watercress.

NOTE Almost the entire U.S. hazelnut crop is grown in Oregon by only 650 farms on nearly 30,000 acres. Hazelnuts are unique for two very important reasons: first, they're the tree nut that is highest in folate, a very important nutrient, particularly for women who are pregnant or may become pregnant. More interesting to me, hazelnuts are unique in that they pollinate in the middle of winter and stay dormant until the weather improves, as opposed to pollinating in early spring the way most other trees do.

NUTRITION INFORMATION: SERVING SIZE: 3–4 pieces of tofu • CALORIES: 460 • CALORIES FROM FAT: 340 • TOTAL FAT: 38 grams • SATURATED FAT: 4.5 grams • CHOLESTEROL: 95 milligrams • SODIUM: 85 milligrams • TOTAL CARBOHYDRATE: 15 grams • FIBER: 5 grams • PROTEIN: 20 grams

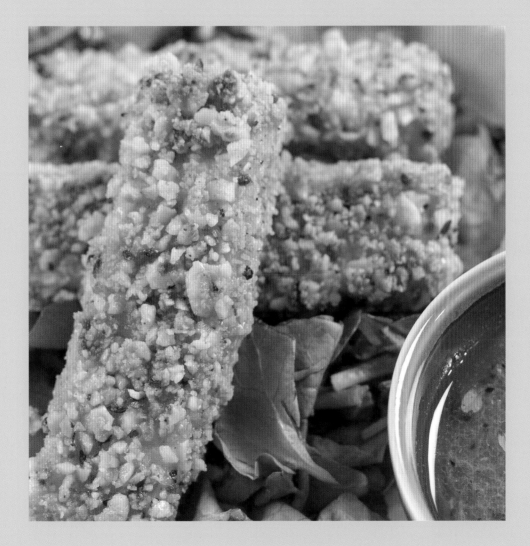

Oven-Fried Chicken and Waffles
with Blueberry Compote

I use the term "fried" very loosely here. "Waffles," too. I don't have my own waffle iron, so sometimes when I've made this recipe, it's been closer to chicken and pancakes—and still delicious. But I must admit that the waffle iron adds an airiness to the batter that I've been unable to replicate with just a pan. Though the chicken is baked, Chex cereal gives it a satisfying crunch, and the coating is thick enough to ensure the chicken's juiciness.

Serves 6

Chicken

- ⅓ cup all-purpose flour
- Salt and freshly ground black pepper
- 2 eggs
- ¼ cup water
- 1½ cups Wheat Chex
- ¼ cup chopped fresh thyme leaves
- 6 boneless, skinless chicken breasts (can also use bone-in breasts, but cooking time will be increased)

To make the chicken, preheat the oven to 350°F. Sprinkle the flour on a large plate and season with salt and pepper. In a shallow bowl, beat together the egg and water. Crush the cereal and mix it together with the chopped thyme in another shallow bowl. Rinse the chicken and pat dry. Working with one chicken breast at a time, dredge it in the flour, shaking off the excess, and then dip it in the egg mixture and then in the crushed cereal, making sure it's fully coated. Place the coated chicken on a baking sheet that has been lightly sprayed with olive oil. Repeat with the remaining chicken breasts.

Bake the chicken until it is golden and crisp and a meat thermometer inserted into the center registers 170°F, about 20 minutes.

To make the compote, combine the blueberries, maple syrup, and maple extract in a small saucepan. Cook over medium-low heat until most of the berries have burst and the mixture has begun to thicken, about 10 minutes.

While the chicken and the compote cook, make the waffles (do this step last so that the waffles are eaten immediately). Heat up a waffle iron. Beat the egg whites until they form stiff peaks; set aside. Mix together the egg yolks, milk, and vegetable oil in a medium-size bowl. In a large bowl, combine the flour, baking powder, baking soda, and salt. Add the wet ingredients to the dry ingredients and mix until combined and then gently fold in the egg whites. Let the batter rest 10 minutes and then cook the waffles one at a time, according to the manufacturer's directions.

Serve each chicken breast with a waffle, drizzled with 1 tablespoon blueberry compote.

Compote

- 1 pint blueberries
- 2 tablespoons maple syrup
- ½ teaspoon maple extract

Waffles

- 2 eggs, separated
- 1⅓ cups skim milk
- ¼ cup vegetable oil
- ¾ cup whole-wheat pastry flour
- 2 teaspoons baking powder
- ¼ teaspoon baking soda
- ¼ teaspoon salt

NOTE Pastry flour is a low-gluten flour used to make batters that should be light and fluffy. Whole-wheat pastry flour is lighter and softer than regular whole-wheat flour and healthier than its white counterpart. It is a little bit heavier (flavorwise) than white pastry flour, making it ideal for savory waffles or baked goods.

NUTRITION INFORMATION: SERVING SIZE: 1 chicken breast, 1 waffle, 1 tablespoon compote • CALORIES: 460 • CALORIES FROM FAT: 140 • TOTAL FAT: 16 grams • SATURATED FAT: 3 grams • CHOLESTEROL: 200 milligrams • SODIUM: 540 milligrams • TOTAL CARBOHYDRATE: 44 grams • FIBER: 5 grams • PROTEIN: 35 grams

Braised Shrimp
in Tomatillo-Pepitas Sauce

Most tomatillo and pumpkin seed (*pepitas*) sauces call for unnecessary sugar or honey; omitting them still results in a creamy but hearty sauce. Here the shrimp is cooked in the freshly made sauce, where it absorbs all the rich, nutty flavor.

Serves 4

1 tablespoon olive oil

1 white onion, chopped

3 cloves garlic, halved

15 tomatillos, husked and quartered

1 jalapeño, seeded and quartered

1½ cups low-sodium chicken broth

1½ cups green pumpkin seeds, roasted but not salted*

1 dried chile de árbol (can omit or add more cayenne instead of chile de árbol)

1 teaspoon ground cumin

½ teaspoon paprika

Pinch of cayenne

Salt and freshly ground black pepper

1½ pounds shrimp, peeled and deveined

Preheat the oven to 350°F. Heat the oil in a cast iron pan over medium heat. Add the onions and garlic and cook for 2 minutes. Add the tomatillos and jalapeño and cook for 3 minutes. Transfer the pan to the oven and roast for 35–40 minutes, stirring every 15 minutes.

Scrape the tomatillo mixture into a food processor, along with the chicken broth, pumpkin seeds, chile de árbol, cumin, paprika, cayenne, and salt and pepper to taste. Blend until the mixture is very smooth.

Pour the mixture back into the cast iron pan and bring to a simmer over low heat. Add the shrimp and cook, stirring occasionally, until pink and cooked through, 3–5 minutes.

If you want to roast the pumpkin seeds yourself, purchase raw green pumpkin seeds, soak them overnight, and then bake them in a 350°F oven for about 15 minutes, stirring several times throughout the cooking. Stay close to the oven, though; when you hear them start to pop, they're done!

NOTE Pumpkin seeds are high in several minerals, such as magnesium and zinc. Some early research suggests that pumpkin seeds may play a positive role in preventing complications for people with diabetes (more research is underway).

NUTRITION INFORMATION: SERVING SIZE: 1 cup sauce and 8–10 shrimp per person (depending on size) • CALORIES: 320 • CALORIES FROM FAT: 100 • TOTAL FAT: 11 grams • SATURATED FAT: 1.5 grams • CHOLESTEROL: 215 milligrams • SODIUM: 650 milligrams • TOTAL CARBOHYDRATE: 27 grams • FIBER: 8 grams • PROTEIN: 30 grams

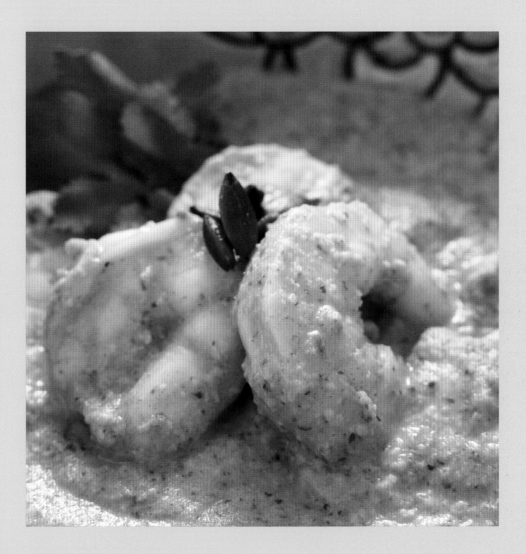

Spicy Crusted Flounder
with a Plum Salsa

Through most of my life, including my adult life, it never occurred to me that I could make salsa with fruits other than peaches, mangoes, or tomatoes. Those are the standard choices but certainly not the end-all, be-all of salsa ingredients. When plums are in season, choose a colorful variety to use in the salsa to give this recipe an extra punch of color (and nutrients).

Serves 4

4 plums, preferably a mix of red, purple, and yellow varieties, pitted and diced

½ cup diced cucumber

½ cup diced red onion

3 tablespoons chopped cilantro leaves

3 tablespoons freshly squeezed lime juice

1 small jalapeño, seeded and finely minced

1 clove garlic, finely minced

1 tablespoon olive oil

Salt and freshly ground black pepper

½ cup buttermilk

½ cup corn flour (masa harina)

1 tablespoon dried oregano

1½ teaspoons ground cumin

1½ teaspoons ground ginger

1 teaspoon cayenne (¾ teaspoon if you don't want it too spicy)

4 (6-ounce) flounder fillets, deboned and cleaned

To make the salsa, combine the plums, cucumber, red onion, cilantro, lime juice, jalapeño, garlic, and olive oil in a bowl and mix well; season to taste with salt and pepper. Refrigerate, covered, to let the flavors blend.

Preheat the broiler and place a rack 4–6 inches below the heating element. Lightly spray a baking sheet with olive oil or another cooking spray to prevent sticking. Pour the buttermilk in a wide, shallow bowl. In another shallow bowl, mix together the corn flour, oregano, cumin, ginger, and cayenne; season to taste with salt and pepper.

Dip one fish fillet in buttermilk, letting the excess drip off. Dredge it in the corn flour mixture, making sure that it is well coated. Place the fillet on the baking sheet and repeat with the other fillets. Lightly spray the coated fillets with olive oil. Broil the fillets, flipping halfway through, until the flesh flakes with a fork, 3–4 minutes per side.

Serve the fish with the plum salsa.

NOTE Plums, along with their dried counterpart (prunes), have a unique set of antioxidants, including a high content of vitamin C. They also contain a good dose of vitamin K and potassium, assisting in reducing blood pressure and lowering the risk of stroke. Remember to eat the skin; it's where a lot of the vitamins and fiber are.

NUTRITION INFORMATION: SERVING SIZE: 1 fillet plus about ¼ cup salsa • CALORIES: 330 • CALORIES FROM FAT: 100 • TOTAL FAT: 11 grams • SATURATED FAT: 2 grams • CHOLESTEROL: 110 milligrams • SODIUM: 760 milligrams • TOTAL CARBOHYDRATE: 23 grams • FIBER: 3 grams • PROTEIN: 34 grams

Summer Quinoa Casserole
with Snow Peas

This is not your typical casserole. Instead of being laden with canned cream of mushroom soup, gluey pasta, and overcooked vegetables, this fresh casserole features crisp snow peas and quinoa. Although this recipe is a simple summer version, you can tailor the flavors to whatever is currently in season. If I were making this in autumn, I might use broccoli and mushrooms. I encourage you to try making it with your favorite vegetable combinations.

Serves 6

3 cups low-sodium chicken broth

1 cup quinoa

1 tablespoon olive oil

4 shallots, sliced

2 cloves garlic, minced

4 cups chopped arugula

8 ounces snow peas, roughly chopped

1 cup shredded Dubliner cheese

Salt and freshly ground black pepper

Preheat the oven to 375°F. Combine the chicken broth and quinoa in a medium-size pot and bring to a boil. Reduce the heat and simmer until the quinoa is tender, about 15 minutes.

Meanwhile, heat the olive oil in a medium-size pan over medium heat. Add the shallots and cook, stirring occasionally, until lightly caramelized, about 15 minutes. Add the garlic and cook until fragrant, 2–3 minutes more.

Lightly spray an 11 × 7–inch pan with olive oil. Drain the quinoa (if there is extra liquid in the pan) and toss with the shallot mixture, arugula, snow peas, Dubliner cheese, and salt and pepper. Spread evenly in the pan and bake until lightly browned, 25–30 minutes.

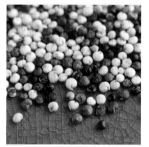

NOTE Quinoa has become very trendy in recent years and is unique because it is a complete protein (which we often think comes only from animal sources). However, consuming a reasonable portion size adds a little protein but not all that much. The biggest benefit is that because it's so high in protein, it's lower in carbohydrate than many other grains.

NUTRITION INFORMATION: SERVING SIZE: 1 cup • CALORIES: 250 • CALORIES FROM FAT: 90 • TOTAL FAT: 10 grams • SATURATED FAT: 4.5 grams • CHOLESTEROL: 20 milligrams • SODIUM: 160 milligrams • TOTAL CARBOHYDRATE: 28 grams • FIBER: 3 grams • PROTEIN: 12 grams

Greek-Style Fish Tacos
with Crunchy Garbanzos

Tacos are delicious in any form, but fish tacos are too often fried and any freshness is left up to cabbage—a weak afterthought, in my opinion. This crisp garbanzo bean topping gives you some crunch to add on top, and you'll probably have leftovers for snacks.

Serves 4

½ cup pine nuts

15–20 large basil leaves

3 cloves garlic

⅓ cup olive oil

1½ pounds cod

1 (15-ounce) can garbanzo beans, rinsed and drained

1 teaspoon ground cumin

½ teaspoon paprika

¼ teaspoon garlic powder

Salt and freshly ground black pepper

8 corn tortillas, warmed

15–20 Kalamata olives, pitted and chopped

10–15 grape tomatoes, quartered

Small handful of fresh parsley leaves, chopped

4 ounces feta cheese

1 lemon, cut into wedges

Combine the pine nuts, basil, and garlic in a food processor. With the machine running, slowly add the olive oil and blend until combined and smooth. Spread the pesto evenly over the cod and refrigerate, covered, for 30–60 minutes to marinate.

Meanwhile, preheat the oven to 400°F. Toss the garbanzo beans with the cumin, paprika, and garlic powder; season to taste with salt and pepper. Lightly spray the beans with olive oil and spread in one layer in a roasting pan. Roast, stirring often, until the beans are crunchy, 8–10 minutes. Once the roasted garbanzo beans have cooled, chop about ¼ cup of them for sprinkling on the tacos. Save the remaining garbanzo beans for a snack.

Roast the cod until a meat thermometer inserted into the center of the fish registers 145°F, about 15 minutes. Cut the cod into eight equal pieces and fold into the warm tortillas. Top each taco with some olives, tomatoes, and parsley. Sprinkle 1 tablespoon chopped crunchy garbanzo beans and ½ ounce feta cheese over each taco. Serve with the lemon wedges.

NOTE Chickpeas are a great source of protein, fiber, and iron. Canned chickpeas and dry chickpeas are very different in their carbohydrate content: dry chickpeas that you cook yourself have about 6 grams less carbohydrate than canned chickpeas (in a half cup serving). Though I analyzed this recipe using canned chickpeas (to be conservative about their impact on blood sugar), use dry whenever possible.

NUTRITION INFORMATION: SERVING SIZE: 2 tacos • CALORIES: 630 • CALORIES FROM FAT: 350 • TOTAL FAT: 37 grams • SATURATED FAT: 4 grams • CHOLESTEROL: 75 milligrams • SODIUM: 470 milligrams • TOTAL CARBOHYDRATE: 39 grams • FIBER: 5 grams • PROTEIN: 37 grams

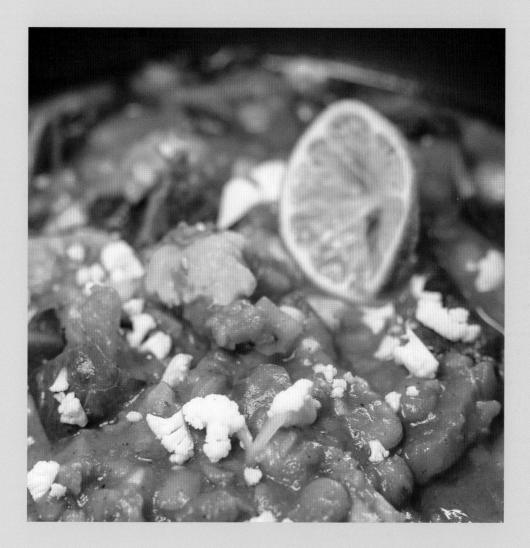

Smoked Gouda and
Broccoli Lasagnettes

One of the things I love about lasagna is just how many different combinations of ingredients—meats, cheeses, herbs, spices, and sauce—can be used to make a delicious dish. One of the things I don't like about lasagna is that it's really easy to overeat. A quick and easy way to preportion your meals is by making what I call lasagnettes—mini lasagnas made in a muffin tin. When they are made with wontons instead of pasta, you can save on carbohydrates and calories. They're also easy to grab as an on-the-go snack, they travel well, and they're perfect for freezing individually for future meals.

Serves 6

36 round wonton wrappers
Olive oil spray
2 cups finely shaved broccoli
2 handfuls spinach, chopped
1½ cups shredded smoked Gouda
½ Vidalia onion, finely chopped
4 garlic cloves, minced
Leaves from 3 sprigs fresh thyme
Pinch of crushed red pepper
Salt and freshly ground black pepper

Preheat the oven to 350°F. Create a workstation with all the ingredients in prep bowls in front of you. Lightly spray a muffin tin with olive oil and place one wonton wrapper at the bottom of each of the cups. Assemble the lasagnettes by adding layers of vegetables, cheese, herbs, spices, and wontons, using up to three wonton layers per muffin cup.

Bake for 20 minutes. Let cool in the pan for a few minutes before serving so that the lasagnettes remain intact; if you take them out too soon, they'll be a gooey (but delicious) mess.

NOTE We all know how healthy broccoli can be, but what you may not know is that a particular compound in broccoli acts as an antioxidant and also shows promise in helping lessen the negative effects of diabetes.

INFORMATION: SERVING SIZE: 2 lasagnettes • CALORIES: 200 • CALORIES FROM FAT: 60 • TOTAL FAT: 7 grams • SATURATED FAT: 4 grams • CHOLESTEROL: 25 milligrams • SODIUM: 390 milligrams • TOTAL CARBOHYDRATE: 23 grams • FIBER: 2 grams • PROTEIN: 10 grams

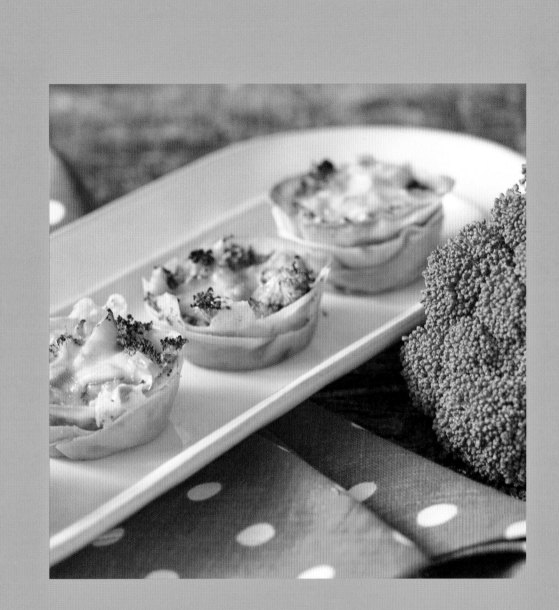

Autumn Tomato Soup
and Baked Apple and Cheddar Gallete

A grilled cheese sandwich is always delicious. What's not to like? Butter, cheese, bread—yes, please! But it's meant to be a treat, not an everyday meal. This recipe takes the best parts of a grilled cheese sandwich and makes them healthy enough to enjoy daily. By losing the bread, we lose carbohydrates, and by pairing the gallette with a vegetable soup, we give this cheese concoction a bigger nutritional punch.

Serves 6

1 head elephant garlic

3 teaspoons olive oil, divided

10 plum tomatoes, halved

½ Vidalia onion, chopped

2 sprigs rosemary leaves, chopped

1 cup low-sodium chicken broth

Salt and freshly ground black pepper

9 phyllo dough sheets

2 Granny Smith apples, thinly sliced

12 ounces sharp white cheddar cheese, thinly sliced

To make the soup, preheat the oven to 350°F. Cut off the top of the head of garlic, exposing the cloves; drizzle 1 teaspoon olive oil over top and wrap in foil. Put the tomatoes in a roasting pan and toss with the remaining 2 teaspoons olive oil. Put the garlic and the pan of tomatoes in the oven and roast for 1 hour.

When the garlic cloves are cool enough to handle, pop them from their papery husks and transfer to a blender or food processor, along with the roasted tomatoes, onion, rosemary, and chicken broth. Puree until smooth and then transfer the mixture to a pot and simmer, covered, over low heat for 30 minutes. Remove the lid, season with salt and pepper, and simmer for 15 minutes more.

While the soup simmers, make the cheddar galette. Preheat the oven to 375°F. Lay a sheet of phyllo on a cutting board, spray with olive oil, and repeat with the other two sheets. Using anything about 6 inches in diameter as a guide, cut six 6-inch circle of layered phyllo. Place a circle of phyllo on the baking sheet and arrange ⅙ of the apple slices in a pinwheel. Sprinkle with ⅙ of the cheese, and fold the phyllo edges over the outer edge of the apples. Repeat with the other 5 circles of phyllo, spacing them on the baking sheet so that they don't touch. Bake until the cheese is melted and the phyllo is golden, about 20 minutes.

NOTE There are hundreds of varieties of tomatoes, and they come in many colors, shapes, and sizes. It was first thought that only red tomatoes contain the antioxidant lycopene, but it turns out that orange tomatoes also have a lot of the health-protective phytonutrient.

NUTRITION INFORMATION: SERVING SIZE: 1 grilled cheese and 1 cup soup • CALORIES: 400 • CALORIES FROM FAT: 220 • TOTAL FAT: 24 grams • SATURATED FAT: 13 grams • CHOLESTEROL: 60 milligrams • SODIUM: 490 milligrams • TOTAL CARBOHYDRATE: 29 grams • FIBER: 4 grams • PROTEIN: 15 grams

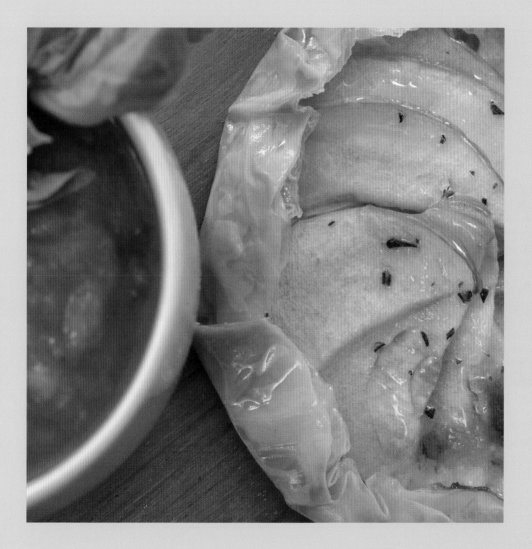

Farmhouse Salad
with a Poached Egg

When I think of a hearty vegetarian meal, I think of a meal that is bright, flavorful, and filling. This recipe—chewy, crisp, colorful, and rich without being laden with calories—is the physical manifestation of that ideal. I made this recipe for my brother and sister-in-law, and they have subsequently made it many times with whatever seasonal vegetables they have on hand. It's so versatile that maybe it should be called a kitchen sink salad!

Serves 6

3 cups low-sodium chicken stock

1 cup wheatberries

6 bell peppers, preferably a mix of red, orange, and yellow, roughly chopped

1 pound mushrooms, trimmed and quartered

1 Vidalia onion, sliced

1 bunch kale, roughly chopped

½ cup pine nuts

15–20 large basil leaves

¼ cup grated pecorino cheese

3 cloves garlic

⅓ cup olive oil

6 eggs

3 tablespoons white vinegar

Bring the chicken stock to a boil in a medium-size pot and add the wheatberries. Simmer, covered, until al dente, about 30 minutes. Remove from the heat and drain off any remaining liquid. Set the wheatberries aside.

Preheat the oven to 425°F. Place the peppers and mushrooms on baking sheets and spray lightly with olive oil. Roast until browned and tender, about 20 minutes. Transfer to plates so that you can use the baking sheets again.

Place the onion on a baking sheet, spray lightly with olive oil, and roast until golden and tender, about 30 minutes. Place the kale on a baking sheet, spray lightly with olive oil, and roast for about 5 minutes.

While the vegetables are roasting, toast the pine nuts in a dry skillet over medium-low heat, stirring often, until golden brown, 5–6 minutes. Remove from the heat.

In a food processor or blender, pulse the pine nuts, basil, pecorino, and garlic. With the motor running, add the olive oil in a slow stream and blend until combined.

To assemble the salad, toss the wheatberries with the vegetables. Fill a medium-size saucepan with 1–1½ inches of water and add the vinegar. Bring the mixture to a boil. Gently crack three eggs into the water, remove from heat, and slowly stir the water. Let the eggs sit for about 5 minutes. Remove with a slotted spoon. Repeat with the remaining eggs. Top each salad with 1–2 teaspoons of pesto and a poached egg. Serve immediately.

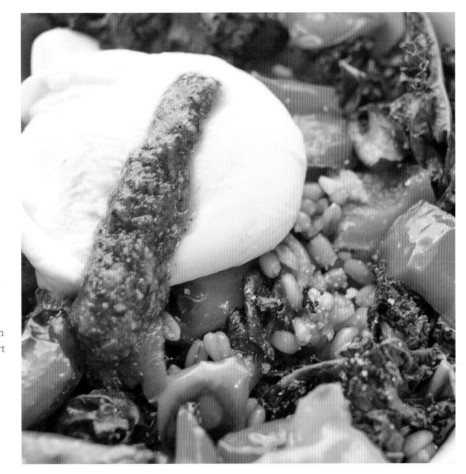

NOTE Eggs (particularly the yolks) once were condemned for their cholesterol content, but the yolks contain omega-3 fats and are great sources of vitamin B_{12}, choline, and selenium. Although the verdict is still out on how much risk the cholesterol in eggs poses, they can be part of a healthy diet.

NUTRITION INFORMATION: SERVING SIZE: ⅓ cup wheatberries, 1 cup vegetables, 1 egg • CALORIES: 480 • CALORIES FROM FAT: 240 • TOTAL FAT: 27 grams • SATURATED FAT: 5 grams • CHOLESTEROL: 190 milligrams • SODIUM: 220 milligrams • TOTAL CARBOHYDRATE: 41 grams • FIBER: 7 grams • PROTEIN: 20 grams

Seared Lemon Pepper
Tuna

In my experience, seared tuna often is coated with sesame seeds, usually both white and black, making a very delicious piece of fish but one we've all seen on menu after menu. This is a different take with less fat but, I think, more kick. Coating the tuna in lemon juice begins to "cook" the fish before it hits the pan, making the cooking time even shorter. Don't walk away from the stove even for a minute or the tuna will be overcooked and you'll miss the delicateness of a good-quality piece of fish.

Serves 4

- 6 lemons, zested and juiced to yield ¼ cup juice and at least 6 tablespoons zest
- 2–3 tablespoons freshly ground black pepper
- 4 (6-ounce) sushi-grade tuna steaks
- 2 tablespoons olive oil, for spraying

Finely grate the zest from enough lemons to make at least 6 tablespoons. Transfer the zest to a shallow bowl, along with the black pepper. Juice enough lemons to make ¼ cup juice; put the juice in another shallow bowl.

Rinse the tuna and pat dry. Quickly dip a tuna steak in the lemon juice and then coat with the pepper and lemon zest mixture. Repeat with all of the tuna steaks. You might need more lemon zest and pepper if the steaks are thin, with a lot of surface area.

Heat a large cast iron pan over medium-high heat. Lightly spray the pan with the oil, add the steaks, and sear each steak for 2–3 minutes per side (for medium-rare tuna).

NOTE Two teaspoons of black pepper contains more than 10 percent of the recommended daily amount of vitamin K. It also aids digestion by stimulating the stomach to release acids that break down foods. The longer pepper cooks, the more its flavor is lost, so add it toward the end of cooking when possible.

NUTRITION INFORMATION: SERVING SIZE: 1 tuna steak • CALORIES: 330 • CALORIES FROM FAT: 140 • TOTAL FAT: 15 grams • SATURATED FAT: 3 grams • CHOLESTEROL: 65 milligrams • SODIUM: 70 milligrams • TOTAL CARBOHYDRATE: 6 grams • FIBER: 2 grams • PROTEIN: 40 grams

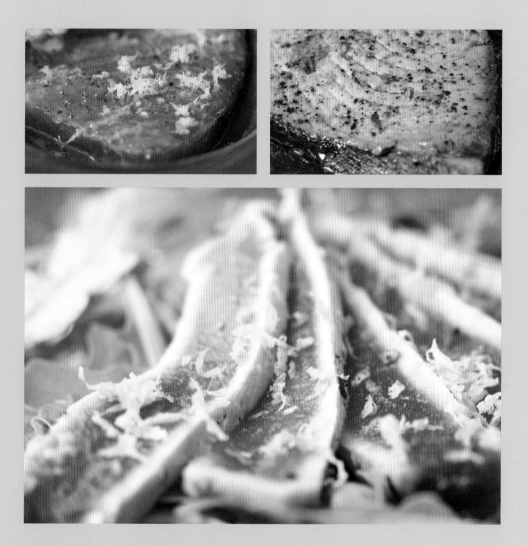

Beet and Black Bean Burger Salad
with Lime-Avocado Dressing

One of the best veggie burgers I ever ate was from a small diner in Manhattan. I asked the waitress if she could find out what was in it. When she returned several minutes later, she walked straight over to my table, handed me a piece of paper, and said, "Well, I have to admit that I'm surprised, but these veggie burgers are prepackaged and frozen! They have an ingredient list on the side of the box, so I wrote down everything." I glanced down at the paper, which must have had 20 or so ingredients, thanked her profusely, and thought, *I am never going to make a burger that requires so much work.* So I set out to make something simpler, and this recipe is the result. The beets add sweetness, which contrasts nicely with the meaty black beans. This burger doesn't need a bun; instead, I like it served on top of the beet greens with a thick, creamy avocado dressing.

Serves 6

Burgers

- 2 large beets, scrubbed
- ¼ cup sunflower seeds
- 1 (15-ounce) can black beans, rinsed and drained
- 1 egg, beaten
- ½ cup oats
- 2 tablespoons chopped fresh oregano leaves
- 1½ teaspoons smoked paprika
- 1 teaspoon ground cumin
- 1 teaspoon ground ginger
- 1 teaspoon garlic powder
- 1 teaspoon onion powder

Preheat the oven to 400°F. Wrap the beets tightly in aluminum foil and roast until tender, 45–60 minutes. When cool enough to handle, peel the beets and grate them.

Preheat a grill to medium-high. Using a mortar and pestle, grind the sunflower seeds until they are mostly ground.

In a large shallow bowl, mash the black beans with a potato masher. When the beans are a little pasty but still include some partially intact beans, add the sunflower seeds, grated beets, egg, oats, oregano, paprika, cumin, ginger, garlic powder, and onion powder. Mix gently until combined. Shape the mixture into six patties.

Lightly oil the grill rack to keep the burgers from sticking. Grill the burgers over medium-high heat for about 6 minutes on each side.

Salad

- 1 avocado, pitted, peeled, and chopped
- 1 tablespoons chopped fresh oregano leaves
- ¼ cup freshly squeezed lime juice
- 2 tablespoons water
- Salt and freshly ground black pepper
- 10 cups chopped beet greens

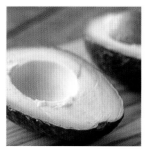

In a blender or food processor, combine the avocado, the remaining tablespoon of oregano, lime juice, and 2 tablespoons water; season to taste with salt and pepper. Blend until smooth, adding more water if you want a thinner dressing. Toss the chopped beet greens with the dressing and divide between six plates. Top the salads with a burger and drizzle any remaining dressing over the burgers.

NOTE Though high in carbohydrates, beets have phytonutrients that no other vegetables have called betalains (which have antioxidant, anti-inflammatory, and detoxification properties). Be careful, though: the longer the beets are cooked, the more betalains you lose, so don't steam them for more than 15 minutes or roast them longer than 1 hour. You can even eat them raw to get the maximum folate content.

NUTRITION INFORMATION: SERVING SIZE: 1 patty and ½ cup greens • CALORIES: 290 • CALORIES FROM FAT: 110 • TOTAL FAT: 13 grams • SATURATED FAT: 2 grams • CHOLESTEROL: 45 milligrams • SODIUM: 570 milligrams • TOTAL CARBOHYDRATE: 33 grams • FIBER: 13 grams • PROTEIN: 13 grams

Grilled Cauliflower Steaks
with a Nutmeg-Cayenne "Cream" Sauce

A roux—a base of equal parts fat and flour that is used to thicken sauces—can be made with oil or butter. For this dish I prefer butter, but feel free to use 1 tablespoon of vegetable oil instead. You'll be surprised what a satisfying entrée cauliflower can make. The grill infuses the "steaks" with deep smoky flavor, and the creamy cayenne-spiked sauce enriches them further.

Serves 4

1 tablespoon butter

2 shallots, finely minced

1 tablespoon all-purpose flour

1 cup skim milk

¾ cup grated Parmesan cheese

½ teaspoon finely grated nutmeg

¼ teaspoon cayenne

Salt and freshly ground black pepper

2 heads cauliflower: green, orange, purple, or white

1 tablespoon olive oil

To make the sauce, heat the butter in a medium-size saucepan over medium heat. Add the shallots and cook, stirring occasionally, until translucent, 3–4 minutes. Add the flour and cook, stirring constantly, for about 1 minute. Whisk in the milk and continue whisking until thickened, about 3 minutes. Whisk in the Parmesan, nutmeg, and cayenne; season to taste with salt and pepper. Keep warm.

Preheat the grill or a grill pan to medium-high. Slice the cauliflower heads lengthwise into ¾-inch-thick steaks. Lightly spray with the olive oil and season with salt and pepper. Grill until grill marks appear and the cauliflower is crisp-tender, about 5 minutes per side. Remove from the heat and serve with the warm sauce.

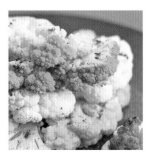

NOTE You might be gasping because I use butter in this recipe, but consider this: (1) a little butter is no worse than any other animal fat, (2) butter has more protein than oil (and less fat per tablespoon), and (3) butter is fairly unprocessed (particularly compared with margarine, even margarine made with nonhydrogenated oil). A former professor, Joan Gussow, who has often been cited for her work in promoting sustainable food systems and organic food, said it best: "As for butter versus margarine, I trust cows more than chemists." Though I personally also trust chemists, I do believe the less processed the food, the better!

NUTRITION INFORMATION: SERVING SIZE: 4 slices cauliflower, 3 tablespoons sauce • CALORIES: 270 • CALORIES FROM FAT: 120 • TOTAL FAT: 14 grams • SATURATED FAT: 7 grams • CHOLESTEROL: 30 milligrams • SODIUM: 460 milligrams • TOTAL CARBOHYDRATE: 20 grams • FIBER: 7 grams • PROTEIN: 18 grams

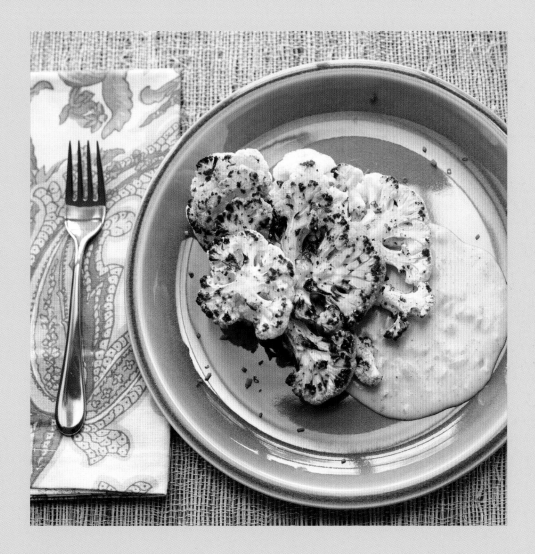

Stuffed Pork Tenderloin
with Mustard-Apple Chutney

The beauty of this dish is in the presentation. Using toothpicks keeps the stuffing inside and creates a beautiful look with very little effort.

Serves 6

¼ cup olive oil

10 sage leaves, finely chopped

1 sprig fresh rosemary, leaves finely chopped

¼ teaspoon garlic powder

Salt and freshly ground black pepper

2 pork tenderloins

2 apples, cored and diced (separated; 1 apple is for the chutney, 1 for the stuffing)

¼ cup low-sodium chicken broth

¼ cup apple cider vinegar

2 tablespoons dried cranberries, chopped

2 tablespoons maple syrup

1 shallot, sliced

3 garlic cloves, chopped, divided

2 tablespoons Dijon mustard

Preheat the oven to 400°F. Stir together the olive oil, sage, rosemary, and garlic powder; season to taste with salt and pepper. Using a sharp knife, butterfly the pork tenderloins by cutting them almost in half lengthwise and opening them like a book. Rub all over with the marinade. Cover and refrigerate for 1 hour.

While the pork marinates, make the chutney. Combine half of the diced apple, the chicken broth, vinegar, cranberries, maple syrup, shallot, and a third of the chopped garlic in a saucepan. Bring to a boil over medium heat and then reduce the heat, cover, and simmer for about 15 minutes. Stir in the mustard and the cornstarch and cook, stirring frequently, for another 5 minutes. Remove from the heat and set aside, covered, to keep warm.

To make the stuffing, heat 1 tablespoon olive oil in a large pan over medium-high heat. Add the spinach, the remaining half of the diced apples, and the remaining two-thirds of the chopped garlic. Cook, stirring occasionally, until the spinach is wilted and the apples are cooked through, 3–4 minutes. Remove from the heat.

Lay the pork open and spread the stuffing evenly over it. Close the pork and secure the sides with wooden toothpicks every 2 inches.

Heat an oven-safe pan over medium heat and spray it lightly with olive oil. Brown the pork on all sides and then transfer it to the oven. Roast until the internal temperature of the meat registers 150°F on a meat thermometer, about 25–30 minutes. Let rest for a few minutes before slicing it between the toothpicks and serving it with the chutney.

1 tablespoon whole-grain
  mustard

1 tablespoon cornstarch

1 tablespoon olive oil

5 ounces baby spinach

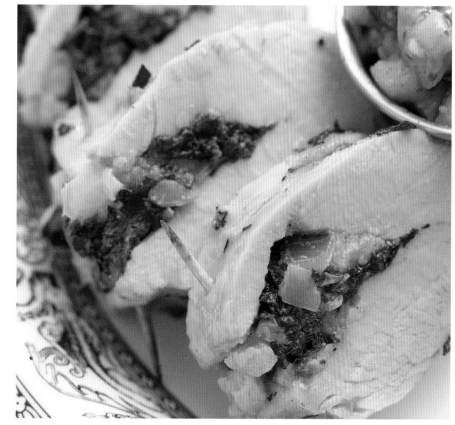

NOTE Ounce for ounce, pork tenderloin has fewer calories, more protein, and less fat than a chicken breast with skin. However, it also has less unsaturated fat and more cholesterol. All in all, pork tenderloin is a pretty healthy choice when grilled, roasted, or broiled.

NUTRITION INFORMATION: SERVING SIZE: 6 ounces pork, 2–3 tablespoons chutney • CALORIES: 300 • CALORIES FROM FAT: 50 • TOTAL FAT: 6 grams • SATURATED FAT: 2 grams • CHOLESTEROL: 100 milligrams • SODIUM: 300 milligrams • TOTAL CARBOHYDRATE: 30 grams • FIBER: 3 grams • PROTEIN: 32 grams.

Rosemary and Mint Marinated Lamb Chops

When I was growing up, my mom always served lamb with bright green mint jelly, which my father loved. But it just seemed a little too, well, processed for me. And when I check the ingredient list, the first item is almost always some form of added sugar (most often high-fructose corn syrup). Lamb is a delicious meat on its own, and though the mint is a very complementary flavor, it doesn't have to come in the form of added sugar.

Serves 4

4 (5- to 6- ounce) bone-in lamb chops

¼ cup balsamic vinegar

¼ cup oil

4 heaping tablespoons finely chopped fresh mint leaves

2 heaping tablespoons chopped fresh rosemary

Preheat a grill to medium-hot. Cut away any excess fat from the lamb chops. Stir together the vinegar, oil, mint, and rosemary and pour over the chops. Cover and refrigerate for at least 1 hour to marinate.

Grill the ribs, turning once, about 3 minutes per side. For a medium-rare chop, the internal temperature should read 120°F while it is on the grill.

NOTE Certain cuts of lamb are just as healthy as lean meats. Since lamb tends to have less marbling than beef, it's actually easier to trim away the fat on fattier cuts. Of course, grilling the meat also helps reduce the fat.

NUTRITION INFORMATION: SERVING SIZE: 1 lamb chop • CALORIES: 160 • CALORIES FROM FAT: 100 • TOTAL FAT: 11 grams • SATURATED FAT: 2.5 grams • CHOLESTEROL: 45 milligrams • SODIUM: 50 milligrams • TOTAL CARBOHYDRATE: 2 grams • FIBER: 1 gram • PROTEIN: 14 grams

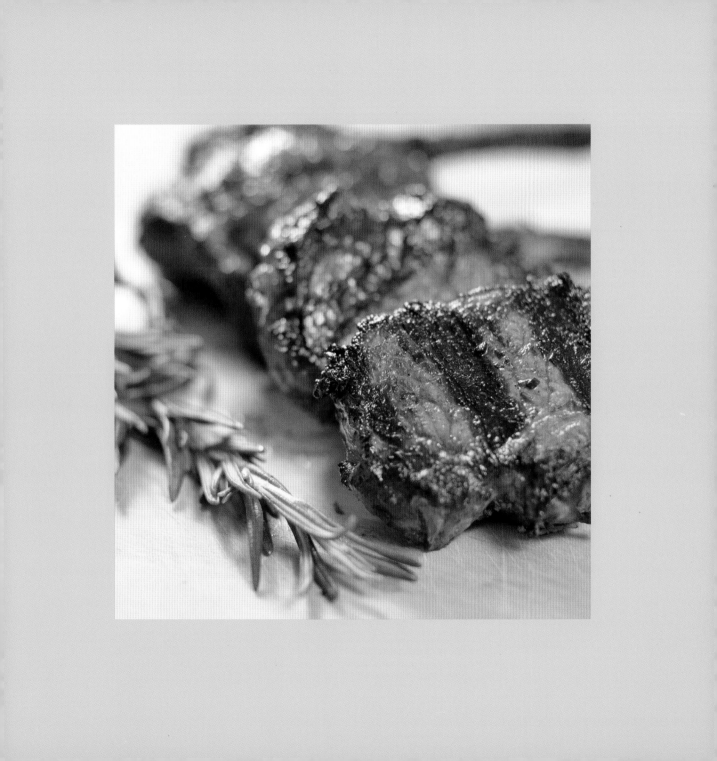

Forty Cloves of Garlic Chicken
with Sweet Potatoes

A classic recipe can always be reimagined and reconstructed. Stuffing herbs and lemon under the skin, along with the garlic, helps build flavor inside and out.

Serves 5–6

2 heads garlic

2 lemons

1 whole chicken (3–4 pounds)

3 medium sweet potatoes, chopped

2 tablespoons olive oil

Salt and freshly ground black pepper

Preheat the oven to 325°F. Separate the garlic cloves and peel about 10 of them. Thinly slice half of the peeled cloves, and slice the remaining 5 in half. Cut 1 of the lemons in half lengthwise, then thinly slice crosswise.

Rinse the chicken and pat it dry. Using your fingers, gently separate the skin from the meat on the breast. Slip the lemon and garlic slices under the skin of the chicken. Fill the cavity of the bird with the unpeeled garlic cloves and the remaining lemon slices. Rub the remaining peeled garlic cloves over the skin of the chicken, reserving the cloves when you're done, and spray the skin lightly with olive oil.

Place the chicken, breast side up, in a roasting pan fitted with a rack. Toss the sweet potatoes and the remaining garlic cloves with the olive oil and scatter around the chicken. Season the chicken and sweet potatoes with salt and pepper. Roast until a meat thermometer registers 165°F and the juices run clear, about 60–80 minutes.

NOTE Eating garlic has long been touted as a preventive measure for a variety of conditions. Primarily, it is known to help prevent heart disease and reduce blood pressure. Others have used it to prevent certain types of cancer and diabetes or to strengthen the immune system, though evidence supporting those claims is less clear.

NUTRITION INFORMATION: SERVING SIZE: 6 ounces chicken without skin • CALORIES: 230 • CALORIES FROM FAT: 70 • TOTAL FAT: 8 grams • SATURATED FAT: 1.5 grams • CHOLESTEROL: 75 milligrams • SODIUM: 120 milligrams • TOTAL CARBOHYDRATE: 13 grams • FIBER: 2 grams • PROTEIN: 24 grams

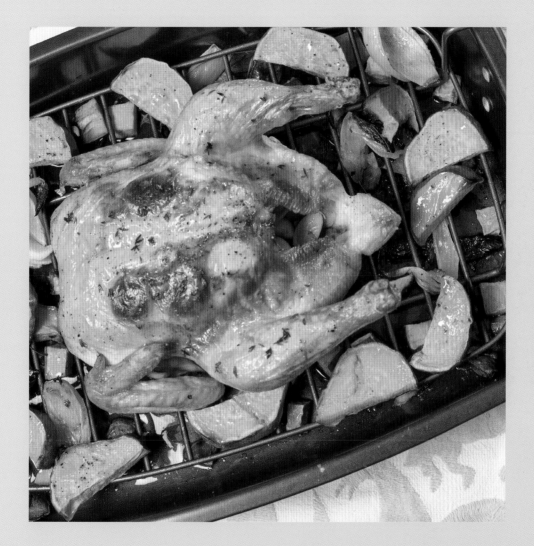

Chipotle Turkey Hash
with Collard Greens

Hash is an "everything but the kitchen sink" kind of meal. It can have meats, eggs, vegetables, grains, cheese—or all of the above! In this winter hash, collard greens and potatoes round out the lean turkey, and the chipotle gives everything some nice heat, like a warming fire in your belly.

Serves: 6

1 tablespoon olive oil

1 medium onion, roughly chopped

3 cloves garlic

2 medium sweet potatoes, diced

1 pound lean ground turkey

5 tablespoons chopped chipotle in adobo

1 tablespoon ground cumin

1 teaspoon paprika

1 teaspoon chili powder

1 bunch collards, chopped (about 6 cups)

Freshly ground black pepper

Heat the olive oil in a large saucepan over medium-high heat. Add the onion and cook, stirring occasionally, until softened and slightly browned, 4–5 minutes. Reduce the heat to medium and add the garlic; cook 2–3 minutes more. Add the sweet potatoes and cook, stirring occasionally, until still slightly firm, 7–8 minutes.

Add the turkey, chipotle, cumin, paprika, and chili powder and cook, stirring frequently, until the turkey is almost cooked through, about 5–6 minutes. Stir in the collard greens, cover, and simmer until the collards are bright green and have softened, 2–3 minutes. Season to taste with pepper. Remove the collard greens from the saucepan with tongs. Place equal-sized portions of greens on 6 plates. Serve topped with turkey hash.

NOTE Chipotles are simply smoked jalapeños. They›re usually available only dried or packed in adobo sauce. Adobo sauce is a spicy tomato sauce made with paprika and a lot of salt (that is why you don't need to add any extra salt to this recipe). You can puree and freeze the remainder of the can (in ice cube trays so that you can easily portion out a tablespoon at a time) or use it in a spicy dip by mixing it into hummus or low-fat cream cheese.

NUTRITION INFORMATION: SERVING SIZE: ¾ cup hash, ½ cup collard greens • CALORIES: 240 • CALORIES FROM FAT: 45 • TOTAL FAT: 5 grams • SATURATED FAT: 0.5 gram • CHOLESTEROL: 45milligrams • SODIUM: 290 milligrams • TOTAL CARBOHYDRATE: 21 grams • FIBER: 5 grams • PROTEIN: 31 grams

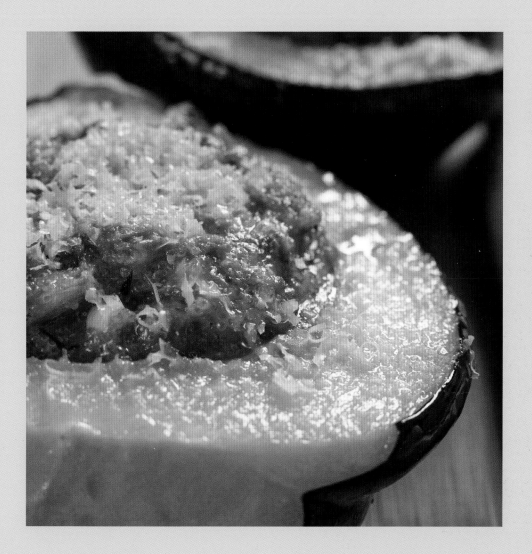

Lean
Shepherd's Pie

An Irish staple, shepherd's pie usually is made with leftover meats and a lot of potatoes. I've completely redesigned the dish, with a healthy twist. Green lentils provide an umami-rich base of flavor, and the roasted and mashed cauliflower and parsnips provide a sweet and savory top layer.

Serves 6

1 medium head cauliflower, chopped into 2-inch florets

1 pound parsnips, chopped into 2-inch pieces

½ cup skim milk

3 tablespoons low-fat cream cheese

Salt and freshly ground black pepper

1 pound lean ground beef

2 tablespoons olive oil, divided

1 pound mushrooms, sliced

3 carrots, chopped

3 stalks celery, chopped

1 leek, chopped

3 garlic cloves, minced

1 cup low-sodium chicken broth

½ cup green lentils

3 tablespoons chopped fresh thyme leaves

1 tablespoon chopped fresh rosemary

Preheat the oven to 425°F. Arrange the cauliflower and parsnips on a baking sheet, spray lightly with olive oil, and roast until they begin to brown, about 25 minutes. Immediately transfer the vegetables to a blender or food processor (to retain some of the moisture), along with the milk and cream cheese; season to taste with salt and pepper. Puree until smooth and set aside. Reduce the oven temperature to 350°F.

Meanwhile, cook the beef, stirring occasionally, in a medium-size pan over medium heat until browned, about 5–6 minutes. Transfer the beef to a bowl.

Using the same pan, heat 1 tablespoon olive oil over medium-high heat. Add the mushrooms and cook, stirring occasionally, until browned, 4–5 minutes. Transfer to the bowl with the beef.

Using the same pan, heat the remaining 1 tablespoon olive oil over medium heat. Add the carrots, celery, leek, and garlic and cook, stirring occasionally, for 3 minutes. Add the chicken broth, lentils, thyme, rosemary, bay leaf, Worcestershire sauce, and cumin. Cover, reduce the heat, and simmer for about 10 minutes. Stir in the flour and cook, uncovered, until it begins to thicken and the lentils are al dente, about 5 minutes. Discard the

1 bay leaf

1 teaspoon
   Worcestershire sauce

½ teaspoon ground cumin

2 tablespoons all-purpose
   flour

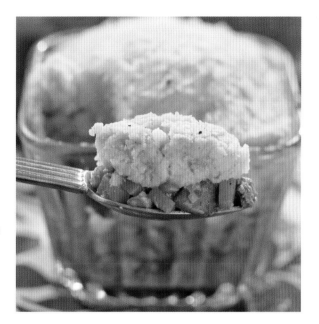

bay leaf and then pour the lentil mixture into the bowl with the beef and mushrooms and stir well to combine.

Spread the beef-lentil mixture evenly in a 9 × 13–inch baking dish. Spread the mashed cauliflower mixture evenly on top. Bake the shepherd's pie until piping hot and golden brown on top, about 20 minutes.

NOTE Parsnip is a root vegetable that is the same shape as a carrot but creamy in color. Smaller parsnips are usually sweeter than large ones. When roasted, they develop a very sweet, tasty flavor unlike that of any other vegetable. Though they're high in sugar like other root vegetables, parsnips are a great ingredient to become familiar with and eat with other, lower-sugar vegetables.

NUTRITION INFORMATION: SERVING SIZE: 1 cup meat mixture, ½ cup mashed vegetables • CALORIES: 310 • CALORIES FROM FAT: 70 • TOTAL FAT: 7 grams • SATURATED FAT: 2 grams • CHOLESTEROL: 45 milligrams • SODIUM: 190 milligrams • TOTAL CARBOHYDRATE: 40 grams • FIBER: 9 grams • PROTEIN: 25 grams

Whole Roasted Trout
with Fennel and Sage

Whole roasted fish is a worthy endeavor because it's really healthy and it doesn't take much effort to make it pack a flavorful punch. The key is to always use aromatics—these are the vegetables, such as onions, carrots, garlic, green pepper, and celery, that are used as a flavor base in many recipes. In this case, I'm using fennel as the flavor builder. The fish traps the flavor and steam inside, cooking while building strong flavors.

Serves 4

4 whole trout, cleaned

1 bulb fennel, thinly sliced

10 fresh sage leaves, thinly sliced

Salt and freshly ground black pepper

Olive oil, for spraying

Preheat the oven to 425°F. Line a baking sheet with parchment paper (use two baking sheets if the fish are very large).

Arrange the trout on the baking sheet and place a few slices of fennel and about ½–1 tablespoon sage inside each fish. Season with salt and pepper and lightly spray the outside of the trout with olive oil. Roast until the flesh is opaque and a meat thermometer inserted into the center of the fish registers 145°F, 15–18 minutes.

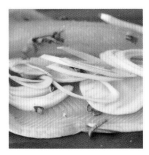

NOTE Chiffonade is a technique used to cut herbs (or leafy vegetables) into long thin strips. The best way to do it is to layer the leaves, roll them up like a cigar, and then slice the cigar crosswise. If you don't want to chiffonade your sage, chopping will work just fine!

NUTRITION INFORMATION: SERVING SIZE: 1 trout • CALORIES: 360 • CALORIES FROM FAT: 120 • TOTAL FAT: 14 grams • SATURATED FAT: 3.5 grams • CHOLESTEROL: 265 milligrams • SODIUM: 200 milligrams • TOTAL CARBOHYDRATE: 3 grams • FIBER: 1 gram • PROTEIN: 54 grams

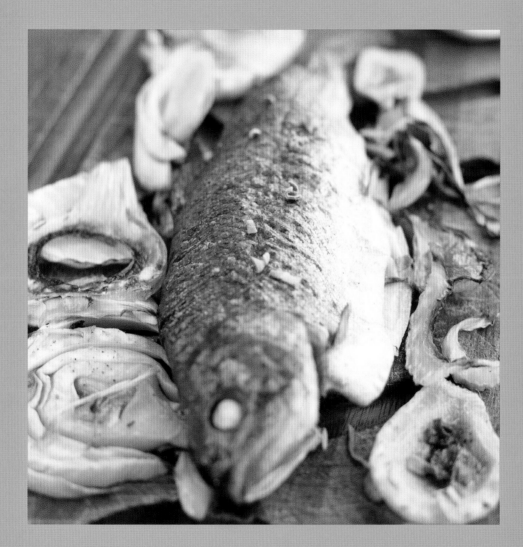

Roasted Poblano Peppers
with BBQ Pulled Chicken

Although barbecue sauce is typically high in sugar, preservatives, and extra stuff, it doesn't have to be off limits. The key to enjoying a homemade barbecue sauce is portion size; luckily, a little bit goes a long way. This recipe makes extra, so use it wisely (try putting it on the lentil loaf, page 90).

Serves 6

1 (14.5-ounce) can low-sodium tomato puree

¾ cup ketchup

⅓ cup apple cider vinegar

⅓ cup light brown sugar

¼ cup Worcestershire sauce

3 tablespoons whole-grain mustard

2 tablespoons freshly squeezed lemon juice

2 tablespoons molasses

2 teaspoons chili powder

2 teaspoons ancho chili powder

1 teaspoon ground horseradish

2 tablespoons vegetable oil

1 small yellow onion, minced

½ green bell pepper, minced

3 cloves garlic, minced

2 tablespoons good-quality whiskey (don't go for the cheap stuff!)

In a large bowl, combine the tomato puree, ketchup, vinegar, brown sugar, Worcestershire sauce, mustard, lemon juice, molasses, chili powder, ancho chili powder, and horseradish and mix until combined.

Heat the oil in a large pot over medium-high heat. Add the onion, pepper, and garlic and cook, stirring occasionally, until it begins to soften, 2–3 minutes. Add the whiskey, stirring and scraping to deglaze the pan. Add the reserved sauce mixture, season with freshly ground black pepper, and bring to a boil. Reduce the heat to low, cover, and cook for about 30 minutes.

Add the chicken breasts and simmer, uncovered, until the chicken is tender and cooked through, about 15 minutes. Taste the sauce and season with salt or pepper if needed.

Meanwhile, preheat the broiler. Cut the poblanos in half lengthwise, discarding the stems and seeds. Arrange, skin side up, in a single layer on a baking sheet. Spray lightly with olive oil and broil for about 3 minutes. Flip the peppers and broil for another 2 minutes.

Preheat the oven to 350°F. Remove the chicken from the sauce and transfer to a work surface. Using two forks, shred the chicken into bite-size pieces. Place the shredded chicken in a bowl and ladle enough sauce on top to keep the chicken moist and hot without drowning it. Set aside the remaining sauce.

Salt and freshly ground
black pepper

4 boneless, skinless
chicken breasts

6 poblano peppers

1 small bunch of cilantro,
chopped

1½ cups shredded sharp
cheddar cheese

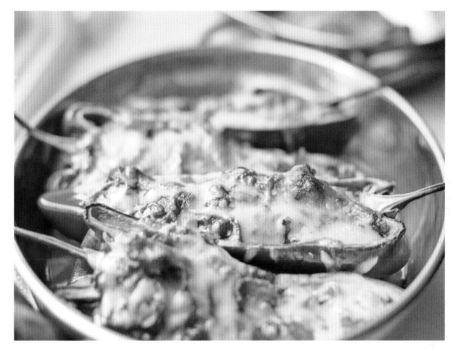

Fill the peppers with shredded chicken. Sprinkle each pepper half with 1 tablespoon cilantro and 2 tablespoons cheddar cheese. Bake until the cheese is melted and starting to bubble, 10–15 minutes. Serve with the remaining cilantro and extra sauce.

NOTE Many barbecue sauces add a lot of sugar, molasses, or ketchup to increase the sweetness, but the calories and sugar add up quickly. If you use low-sodium tomato puree as a base for your sauce, it will have far less sugar. Plus, barbecue sauce doesn't have to be sugary sweet to be delicious.

NUTRITION INFORMATION: SERVING SIZE: 2 pepper halves • CALORIES: 370 • CALORIES FROM FAT: 120 • TOTAL FAT: 13 grams • SATURATED FAT: 5 grams • CHOLESTEROL: 70 milligrams • SODIUM: 730 milligrams • TOTAL CARBOHYDRATE: 35 grams • FIBER: 4 grams • PROTEIN: 26 grams

Braised Chocolate
Mole Chicken

After years of working at New York City farmers' markets, I became good friends with a Mexican family that farmed in New York but lived much of the year in Texas. Toward the end of every summer, the Rodriguez children would head back to Texas with their grandmother while their parents, Maritza and Pedro, would stay in New York to care for the farm until the end of the farmers' market season. The grandmother wouldn't leave, however, without first preparing the most delicious (and obviously authentic) Mexican dishes. My favorite was her mole sauce, and when writing this cookbook, I had to ask if I could include their family recipe. Although this isn't an exact version (I would never be able to replicate years of cultural history and family tradition), Maritza shared with me the most important ingredients and steps to prepare an authentic mole.

Serves 6

1 (4–5-pound) chicken

2 garlic cloves, peeled

6 dried pasilla chilies (chile negro)

4 dried ancho chilies

2 tablespoons vegetable oil

¾ cup currants

½ cup sesame seeds

1 cinnamon stick

6 whole cloves

1 tablespoon dried thyme

1 tablespoon dried oregano

2 ounces Mexican chocolate or 60 percent cacao chocolate, chopped

Salt and freshly ground black pepper

Put the chicken and garlic in a large stockpot and cover with water. Bring to a boil over medium heat and cook until mostly cooked through, about 30 minutes. Leave it in the water for about 10 minutes, then debone.

Remove the stems and seeds from the pasilla chilies, and stem the ancho chilies. Heat the oil in a medium saucepan over medium heat. Add the chilies and lightly fry, turning once, until toasted, about 2 minutes. Using tongs, transfer chilies to a bowl, cover with hot water, and let sit for 30 minutes.

Add the currants to the chili oil in the pan and lightly fry for about 2 minutes. Remove from the heat and transfer the currants to a food processor or blender.

Toast the sesame seeds in a small saucepan over medium heat until lightly browned, about 5 minutes. Scrape the seeds into the food processor with the currants. Return the pan to medium heat, add the cinnamon stick and cloves, and toast, stirring occasionally, until very fragrant, about 5 minutes. Remove from the heat and add to the food processor.

Add the chilies (and their liquid), thyme and oregano to the food processor and blend all ingredients until smooth.

Transfer the sauce to a large pot and heat over medium-low heat. Ladle broth from the chicken pot a ladle at a time until the sauce is simmering

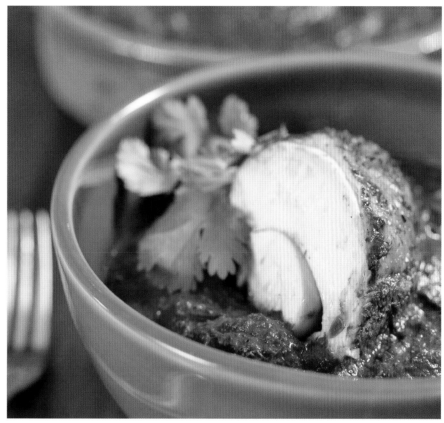

NOTE Mole is a blanket term for many types of Mexican sauces, but they all have chili peppers as a base. Dried chili peppers aren't as easy to come by in the United States as they are in Mexico, and if you're not sure where to get them, ordering online is a great option. Very often, though, supermarkets will have a variety of dried chilies in the ethnic food aisle; for this recipe, I didn't have to go anywhere but my local organic grocery store.

and thick but still pourable, 4–5 cups total. Add the chocolate and stir until melted. Add the chicken, cover with sauce, and simmer for about 20 more minutes, adding more chicken broth if necessary. Discard garlic cloves from the chicken stock. Season with salt and pepper and serve.

NUTRITION INFORMATION: SERVING SIZE: 4–5 ounces chicken meat, about 1½ cups mole • CALORIES: 500 • CALORIES FROM FAT: 180 • TOTAL FAT: 20 grams • SATURATED FAT: 4 grams • CHOLESTEROL: 130 milligrams • SODIUM: 140 milligrams • TOTAL CARBOHYDRATE: 29 grams • FIBER: 7 grams • PROTEIN: 52 grams

Turkey
"Osso Bucco"

By treating the turkey in this recipe the same way you treat the veal when you make osso bucco, you can achieve the same fall-off-the-bone, melt-in-your-mouth texture.

Serves 4

2 tablespoons olive oil

2 pounds bone-in turkey breast (cut in 4 pieces)

1⅓ ounces pancetta, chopped

5 stalks celery, roughly chopped

3 leeks, roughly chopped

3 carrots, roughly chopped

3 cloves garlic, finely chopped

1 cup white wine

1 (28-ounce) can diced San Marzano tomatoes

1 pound button mushrooms, quartered

2 cups low-sodium chicken broth

1½ tablespoons dried juniper berries

5 sprigs fresh rosemary, divided

2 teaspoons dried thyme

1 bay leaf

Heat the olive oil in a large pot over high heat and then add the turkey, skin side down, and cook until golden brown, 5–6 minutes. Transfer the turkey to a plate and set aside.

Reduce the heat to medium. When the pot has cooled down a bit, add the pancetta and cook, stirring occasionally, until browned, about 2 minutes. Add the celery, leeks, carrots, and garlic and cook, stirring occasionally, until the vegetables begin to soften, 5–6 minutes. Add the wine, stirring and scraping the bottom of the pot to deglaze it. Add the tomatoes, mushrooms, chicken broth, juniper berries, 1 sprig whole rosemary, 2 teaspoons thyme, and bay leaf and bring to a simmer. Return the turkey to the pot, cover, and braise for about 90 minutes, stirring occasionally. Let cool in the pot, covered.

Serve one piece of turkey with a ladle of vegetables and broth in a bowl. Garnish with 1 sprig whole rosemary per bowl.

NOTE The technique of braising is a great way to add a lot of flavor to a dish without a lot of calories and fat; it just requires a little extra time and patience. Typically, a braised meat is seared at a high temperature and then cooked in liquid for a long time.

NUTRITION INFORMATION: SERVING SIZE: 6 ounces turkey • CALORIES: 520 • CALORIES FROM FAT: 120 • TOTAL FAT: 14 grams • SATURATED FAT: 2.5 grams • CHOLESTEROL: 75 milligrams • SODIUM: 650 milligrams • TOTAL CARBOHYDRATE: 44 grams • FIBER: 8 grams • PROTEIN: 53 grams

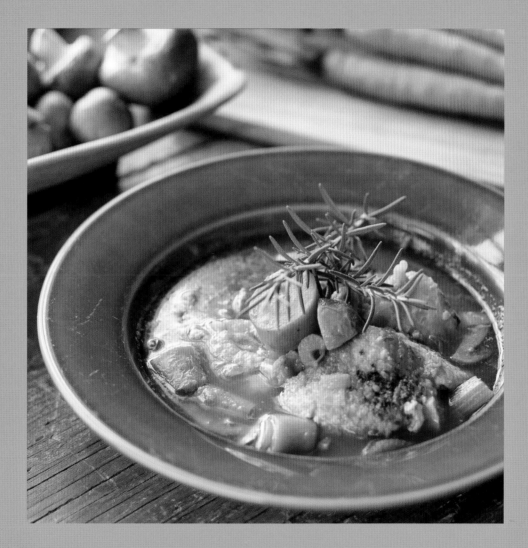

Side Dishes

Side dishes can help complete a meal. If your main dish doesn't have enough vegetables, it will—with these additions! Eating real food using herbs and spices is a great way to create robust flavors and helps you avoid adding carbohydrates or calories to your meals. It doesn't take more than a few minutes—and a full spice rack—to construct savory sides such as Escarole and Beans with Pecorino Cheese and Pecan Pumpkin Tamales.

Balsamic-Glazed Beets
and Garlic Scapes

This recipe is best on a cool spring evening. Cooking the balsamic creates a warming, rich flavor, and the garlic scapes keep it light.

Serves 4

4 medium beets with their greens

2 tablespoons olive oil

1 onion, sliced

3 garlic cloves, minced

¼ cup balsamic vinegar

1 cup chopped garlic scapes

Separate the beets and their greens. Peel and dice the beets; chop the greens, keeping them separate.

Heat the olive oil in a medium-size pot over medium heat. Add the onion and cook, stirring occasionally, until slightly softened, 3–4 minutes. Add the garlic and cook until fragrant, 2–3 minutes. Stir in the diced beets and the vinegar and cook until the beets start to soften, 4–5 minutes. Stir in the scapes and chopped beet greens and cook until most of the vinegar has evaporated and the greens are wilted, about 5 minutes more.

NOTE Garlic scapes—the stalk of the garlic bulb (which is a root)—are a sign of spring. Harvesting the scapes is an easy process; just cut the tops and you're ready to go. If you shop at a farmers' market and they grow garlic but don't sell the scapes, ask the farmers to reserve them for you—chances are, they're throwing the scapes away.

NUTRITION INFORMATION: SERVING SIZE: ½ cup • CALORIES: 130 • CALORIES FROM FAT: 60 • TOTAL FAT: 7 grams • SATURATED FAT: 1 gram • CHOLESTEROL: 0 milligrams • SODIUM: 85 milligrams • TOTAL CARBOHYDRATE: 15 grams • FIBER: 3 grams • PROTEIN: 2 grams

Creamy Asparagus and Farro Salad

This salad is heavy on the vegetables, but the farro adds a nice chewy texture and a lot of fiber. Cream cheese is highly underrated as a dressing ingredient, and it works nicely here.

Serves 6

1 cup farro

2 tablespoons skim milk

3 tablespoons low-fat cream cheese

1 tablespoon olive oil

3 shallots thinly sliced

1 bunch of asparagus, trimmed and roughly chopped

2 ounces pea shoots

4 tablespoons freshly squeezed lemon juice

Finely grated zest of ½ lemon

Salt and pepper to taste

Fill a medium-size pot with about 3 cups of salted water. Add the farro and bring to a boil. Reduce the heat, cover, and simmer until the farro is al dente, 15–20 minutes.

Meanwhile, whisk together the milk and cream cheese in a medium bowl. Set aside.

Heat the olive oil in a medium-size pan over medium heat. Add the shallots and cook, stirring occasionally, until they begin to brown, 2–3 minutes. Add the asparagus and cook, stirring occasionally, until the asparagus is al dente, 3–4 minutes. Remove from the heat.

When the farro is cooked, drain it well and return it to the warm pot. Add the asparagus mixture, cream cheese mixture, pea shoots, lemon juice, and lemon zest. Season to taste with salt and pepper. Mix gently but thoroughly until the farro and asparagus are evenly coated.

NOTE Asparagus is loaded with vitamins such as A, C, E, and K. It's particularly beneficial for people with diabetes because it's also high in chromium, a mineral that improves the functioning of insulin. Another great benefit: it cooks quickly and can be eaten raw. Try shaving raw asparagus with a vegetable peeler for a creative addition to salads.

NUTRITION INFORMATION: SERVING SIZE: ¾ cup • CALORIES: 160 • CALORIES FROM FAT: 40 • TOTAL FAT: 4.5 grams • SATURATED FAT: 1 gram • CHOLESTEROL: 5 milligrams • SODIUM: 40 milligrams • TOTAL CARBOHYDRATE: 27 grams • FIBER: 4 grams • PROTEIN: 6 grams

Sweet and Spicy
Cucumber Salad

This recipe is basically a quick pickle without all the salt and frills. The onion flavor intensifies as the dish sits, so use less than you think you need. Even though they keep well, these cukes are too delicious to last long in your fridge.

Serves 6

½ cup champagne vinegar
2 tablespoons sugar
1 teaspoon salt
1 clove garlic
8 Kirby cucumbers, sliced
½ red onion, finely diced
Crushed red pepper, to taste

Heat the vinegar, sugar, salt, and garlic in a medium-size saucepan over medium heat, stirring, until the sugar dissolves. Combine the cucumbers, red onion, and crushed red pepper in a medium-size bowl. Pour the hot vinegar mixture over the cucumbers and stir until coated evenly. Cover and refrigerate, tossing cucumbers occasionally, for at least 2 hours before serving.

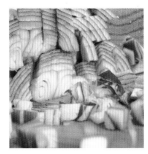

NOTE Many people believe that because cucumbers are so high in water, they have little nutritional value, but that's a myth! One cup of cucumbers meets nearly 20 percent of your daily vitamin K needs in addition to having antioxidants and anti-inflammatory properties. As with most fruits and vegetables, eat the skin for added nutrition.

NUTRITION INFORMATION: SERVING SIZE: ½ cup slices • CALORIES: 35 • CALORIES FROM FAT: 0 • TOTAL FAT: 0 grams • SATURATED FAT: 0 grams • CHOLESTEROL: 0 grams • SODIUM: 50 milligrams • TOTAL CARBOHYDRATE: 10 grams • FIBER: 1 gram • PROTEIN: 5 grams

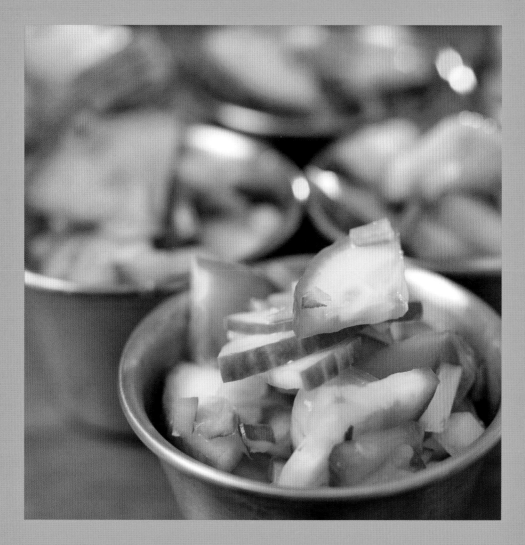

Miso-Marinated
Grilled Summer Squash

There's no question that grilled vegetables are one of the simplest, healthiest summer sides, but I tend to prepare them the same way: marinated in a little balsamic vinaigrette. Though delicious, that preparation gets old. This recipe, seasoned with miso, maximizes the sweet smokiness of grilled vegetables through an entirely different lens.

Serves 4

4 tablespoons rice wine vinegar

3 tablespoons white miso

3 tablespoons water

2 tablespoons low-sodium soy sauce

1 tablespoon sesame oil

4 summer squash, cut lengthwise into ½-inch-thick slices

Whisk together the vinegar, miso, water, soy sauce, and sesame oil in a large bowl. Add the sliced summer squash, toss, and let marinate for 2 hours.

Preheat a grill to medium-high and lightly oil the grill rack. Grill the squash until tender and cooked through, 3–4 minutes per side.

NOTE Miso is a thick paste made from fermented soybeans. In Japan, it comes in many varieties, with flavor profiles ranging from sweet to salty to fruity. The type most typically found in U.S. grocery stores is a sweet white miso that uses rice and barley in combination with soybeans and is very mild.

NUTRITION INFORMATION: SERVING SIZE: 4–5 strips • CALORIES: 70 • CALORIES FROM FAT: 25 • TOTAL FAT: 3 grams • SATURATED FAT: 0 grams • CHOLESTEROL: 0 grams • SODIUM: 420 grams • TOTAL CARBOHYDRATE: 9 grams • FIBER: 2 grams • PROTEIN: 3 grams

Maple Brussels Sprouts
Slaw

The day I realized that Brussels sprouts could be eaten raw was a happy day. I already loved Brussels sprouts, but this realization opened up a new world of salads and slaws. If you don't think you like Brussels sprouts, give this recipe a chance. I promise you'll become a sprout supporter, ready to convert a few people yourself.

Serves 8

12 ounces Brussels sprouts, shredded

1 small Gala apple, grated

½ cup toasted chopped pecans

5 scallions, sliced

¼ cup apple cider vinegar

1½ tablespoons olive oil

1 tablespoon maple syrup

½ tablespoon whole-grain mustard

½ tablespoon Dijon mustard

Combine the Brussels sprouts, apples, pecans, and scallions in a large bowl. Whisk together the remaining ingredients in a small bowl and then pour over the Brussels sprouts mixture and toss well. Cover and refrigerate for at least 1 hour before serving.

NOTE The sulfurous odor that Brussels sprouts (like other cruciferous vegetables, such as broccoli) emit is a result of overcooking, which also results in a loss of nutrients. When eaten raw, however, they are packed with fiber, vitamin C, folate, and antioxidants that help fight cancer. Also, Brussels sprouts consist of nearly 20 percent protein—extremely high compared with other vegetables!

NUTRITION INFORMATION: SERVING SIZE: ½ cup • CALORIES: 160 • CALORIES FROM FAT: 66 • TOTAL FAT: 8 grams • SATURATED FAT: 1 gram • CHOLESTEROL: 0 milligrams • SODIUM: 34 milligrams • TOTAL CARBOHYDRATE: 14 grams • FIBER: 4 grams • PROTEIN: 2 grams

Stuffed Swiss Chard
with Sun-Dried Tomato Quinoa

I consider plants with large leaves, such as Swiss chard, tasty, low-carb vessels for complementary foods. If you don't have Swiss chard, don't worry; this quinoa can stand on its own.

Serves 6

8–10 pieces oil-packed sun-dried tomatoes (reserve the oil), chopped

1 small sweet onion, diced

3 cloves garlic, minced

1 teaspoon paprika

2 cups low-sodium chicken broth

1 cup quinoa, rinsed

½ cup pine nuts

Small handful of fresh basil leaves, roughly chopped

Salt and freshly ground black pepper

1 bunch rainbow Swiss chard (sometimes called Bright Lights)

Olive oil, for drizzling

Heat the oil reserved from the sun-dried tomatoes (about 1 tablespoon) in a medium-size saucepan over medium-high heat. Add the onion and cook, stirring occasionally, until softened, about 5 minutes. Reduce the heat to medium and add the garlic, paprika, and chopped sun-dried tomatoes and cook until fragrant, 2–3 minutes.

Stir in the chicken broth and quinoa and bring to a simmer. Cover and cook until the liquid is absorbed and the quinoa is al dente, about 20 minutes.

Preheat the oven to 350°F and bring a large pot of salted water to a boil.

Toast the pine nuts in a small dry pan over medium-low heat until fragrant. Transfer to a plate to cool.

Once the quinoa is cooked, remove from heat. Stir in the basil and toasted pine nuts; season to taste with salt and pepper.

Blanch the Swiss chard leaves in the boiling water just until softened, about 2 minutes. Drain well and pat dry and then lay 1 leaf on the work surface. Scoop about ⅓ cup of the quinoa mixture onto the leaf and wrap it up like a burrito. Place inside a roasting pan and repeat with the remaining leaves and filling. Lightly spray with olive oil (alternatively, cover lightly with tomato sauce) and roast until hot, about 20 minutes.

NOTE Sun-dried tomatoes have more calories and sugar than regular tomatoes because they've lost their water content (from drying in the sun); however, they retain their nutritional value (vitamin C and lycopene). If you use sun-dried tomatoes preserved in olive oil, don't discard the oil. It can be used in this recipe and others or for salad dressings.

NUTRITION INFORMATION: SERVING SIZE: 1 roll • CALORIES: 253 • CALORIES FROM FAT: 111 • TOTAL FAT: 13 grams • SATURATED FAT: 1 gram • CHOLESTEROL: 0 milligrams • SODIUM: 350 milligrams • TOTAL CARBOHYDRATE: 28 grams • FIBER: 4 grams • PROTEIN: 9 grams

Szechuan-Style
Green Beans

There is an art to high-heat wok sautéing, and it works best with dishes that don't have too many ingredients crowding the pan. The beauty of cooking with high heat is that the food really is just a flash in the pan and in only a few minutes you've got a tasty side dish that seems effortless.

Serves 4

2 teaspoons olive oil

1 pound green beans, trimmed (chopped or left whole)

2 tablespoons chopped garlic

1 tablespoon chopped fresh ginger

½ teaspoon crushed red pepper

3 scallions, sliced

1 tablespoon low-sodium soy sauce

Sesame seeds, for garnish (optional)

Heat the oil in a large skillet over medium-high heat. Add the green beans and cook 1–2 minutes; then add the garlic, ginger, and crushed red pepper. When the green beans begin to get browned in spots, add the scallions and the soy sauce. Toss well and cook until most of the soy sauce has been absorbed, 1–2 minutes.

If you like, garnish with a sprinkling of sesame seeds or extra scallion slices.

NOTE Though green beans are rich in color, we mistakenly don't associate them with high nutrition; however, they have a lot of beta-carotene and when frozen retain about 90 percent of their B vitamins. Haricots verts, a type of string bean, are often more tender, longer, leaner, and pricier. For most cooked recipes, regular green beans are less expensive and a little more desirable because they are hardier and can stand up to brief periods of high heat.

NUTRITION INFORMATION: SERVING SIZE: ½ cup • CALORIES: 68 • CALORIES FROM FAT: 22 • TOTAL FAT: 2 grams • SATURATED FAT: 0 grams • CHOLESTEROL: 0 milligrams • SODIUM: 430 milligrams • TOTAL CARBOHYDRATE: 11 grams • FIBER: 4 grams • PROTEIN: 3 grams

Summer
Vegetable Pinwheel

This is a great dish to prepare with kids because you can make attractive patterns with all the different colors and it is very healthy. Because it uses summer vegetables that have a high water content, this side dish is light but filling.

Serves 8

1 zucchini, bias-sliced crosswise

1 red onion, sliced

1 yellow bell pepper, halved lengthwise and sliced crosswise

1 orange bell pepper, halved lengthwise and sliced crosswise

3 medium ripe tomatoes, sliced

¾ cup grated Parmesan cheese

2 tablespoons chopped fresh thyme

2 tablespoons chopped fresh oregano

Preheat the oven to 425°F. In a 9-inch pie pan, pack the vegetable slices standing up, in an alternating pattern. Sprinkle herbs and cheese between the slices as you go, reserving about ¼ cup Parmesan to sprinkle over the top. Roast for 1 hour or until the tops of the vegetables are golden. Serve as vegetable stacks or fanned out horizontally.

NOTE Compared with the soft, mild, and highly processed commercial version of the cheese, true aged Parmesan is hard, salty, and very, very flavorful. Parmigiano Reggiano cheese comes from a very specific region of Italy where its producers pride themselves on the flavor imparted from the region (the terroir). Of course, other types of Parmesan are also delicious—just be sure to purchase a big chip off a high-quality block as this small splurge is worth every penny.

NUTRITION INFORMATION: SERVING SIZE: 8–10 slices • CALORIES: 100 • CALORIES FROM FAT: 40 • TOTAL FAT: 4.5 grams • SATURATED FAT: 2.5 grams • CHOLESTEROL: 15 milligrams • SODIUM: 210 milligrams • TOTAL CARBOHYDRATE: 11 grams • FIBER: 2 grams • PROTEIN: 6 grams

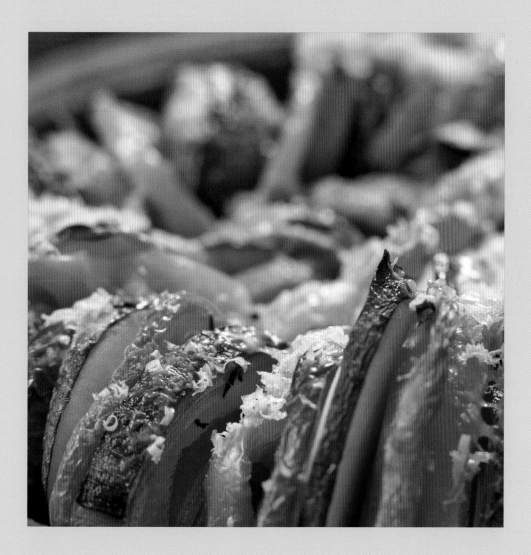

Raw
Jicama Slaw

Jicama is a root vegetable that is light and juicy and makes a great summer slaw. If your arm can make it through all the grating, you'll reap the rewards of a healthier (and tasty) summer slaw.

Serves 8

3 cups julienned or grated jicama

1 cup raw corn kernels

½ cup diced red bell pepper

1 red onion, diced

1 jalapeño, seeded and finely diced

2–3 tablespoons finely chopped fresh cilantro

3 tablespoons lime juice

2 tablespoons olive oil

Salt and freshly ground black pepper

Combine all the ingredients in a bowl and toss well. Cover and chill for at least 1 hour.

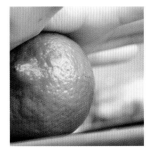

NOTE Jicama is a root vegetable whose brown skin hides a creamy flesh that's mild, watery, and sweet. Like many root vegetables, it is high in starch, but because of its water content, it's not as high in sugar as carrots or beets. Slaw made with jicama is crisp and light. When shopping for jicama, look for firm, heavy ones with thin, unblemished skin.

NUTRITION INFORMATION: SERVING SIZE: ¾ cup • CALORIES: 80 • CALORIES FROM FAT: 33 • TOTAL FAT: 4 grams • SATURATED FAT: 1 gram • CHOLESTEROL: 0 milligrams • SODIUM: 50 milligrams • TOTAL CARBOHYDRATE: 12 grams • FIBER: 3 grams • PROTEIN: 1 gram

Golden Beet and Zucchini Crisps

These crisps are a healthier and more interesting version of potato chips. The cheese becomes golden and hardens the vegetable into a crispy chip. Zucchini has much more water than beets, so make sure to take the time to salt the zucchini slices until they've released much of their moisture.

Serves 4

2 zucchini

¼ cup kosher salt

3 golden beets

1 cup shredded fresh Parmesan

2 tablespoons finely chopped thyme

1½ teaspoons paprika

Salt and freshly ground black pepper

Olive oil, for spraying

Preheat the oven to 450°F. Cut the zucchini on the diagonal into ⅛-inch-thick slices. Place the zucchini in a large colander set in the sink and toss with kosher salt. Let stand for about 10 minutes.

Meanwhile, peel and cut the beets into ⅛-inch-thick slices. Mix together the Parmesan, thyme, and paprika in a small bowl; season to taste with salt and pepper.

Spray two large baking sheets lightly with olive oil. Rinse the zucchini and pat dry. Dip the zucchini pieces in the Parmesan mixture until lightly coated and arrange on the baking sheet. Repeat with the beet slices and the remaining Parmesan mixture. Bake until the vegetables are crisp and the Parmesan is browned, about 25 minutes.

NOTE All beets have iron and fiber, but the yellow color of golden beets means they're also high in vitamins A and C. They also have a milder taste than red beets.

NUTRITION INFORMATION: SERVING SIZE: 4–5 slices total • CALORIES: 150 • CALORIES FROM FAT: 70 • TOTAL FAT: 8 grams • SATURATED FAT: 4.5 grams • CHOLESTEROL: 25 milligrams • SODIUM: 450 milligrams • TOTAL CARBOHYDRATE: 9 grams • FIBER: 2 grams • PROTEIN: 11 grams

Poor Man's Ceviche

As a former vegetarian, I've gotten inspiration from many dishes that aren't plant-based, and ceviche is one of them. This recipe has become a hit at summer cookouts because it's simple and flavorful.

Serves 4

4 summer squash, such as a mixture of zucchini, yellow squash, and pattypan squash

Handful of fresh parsley leaves, roughly chopped

½ cup freshly squeezed lemon juice

¼ cup olive oil

1 clove garlic, grated

¼–½ teaspoon crushed red pepper

Salt and freshly ground black pepper

½ cup crumbled feta or goat cheese

Using a mandoline or vegetable peeler, thinly slice the squash lengthwise. Put the sliced squash in a large bowl (or airtight storage container), along with the parsley.

Whisk together the lemon juice, olive oil, garlic, and crushed red pepper in a small bowl. Pour the dressing over the squash, season with salt and pepper, and toss well. Marinate, covered, in the refrigerator for at least 3 hours and ideally overnight.

Just before serving, add the crumbled feta, season with a little more black pepper, and toss gently.

NOTE Real feta cheese is made in a region of Greece from sheep's or goat's milk. It is creamy, tangy, and salty. Feta, like most other white crumbly cheese, has fewer calories and less fat than hard cheeses such as cheddar. But it is high in carbohydrate and sodium, and so smaller portions are better.

NUTRITION INFORMATION: SERVING SIZE: 1 squash • CALORIES: 200 • CALORIES FROM FAT: 160 • TOTAL FAT: 18 grams • SATURATED FAT: 5 grams • CHOLESTEROL: 15 milligrams • SODIUM: 220 milligrams • TOTAL CARBOHYDRATE: 9 grams • FIBER: 2 grams • PROTEIN: 5 grams

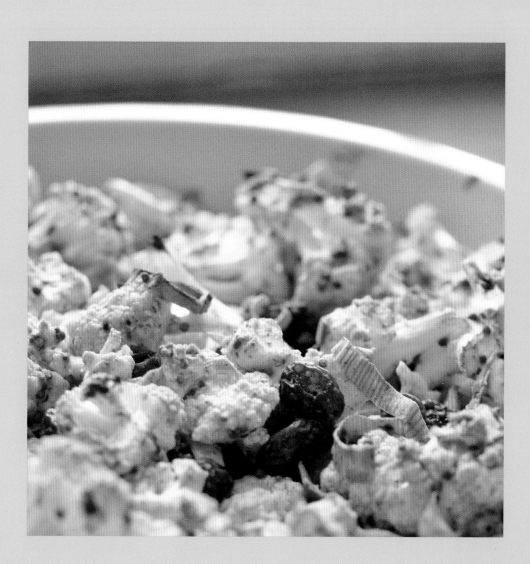

Spiced
Eggplant Rounds

Coating eggplant rounds with spiced yogurt helps them form a crust, almost as if they were deep-fried, but with a subtle smoky aroma and flavor. Let them cool a bit before you take a bite—the outside cools deceptively quickly while the inside remains piping hot and juicy.

Serves 4

1 eggplant

Kosher salt, as needed

½ cup nonfat Greek yogurt

2 teaspoons olive oil

1 teaspoon sweet paprika

½ teaspoon ground cumin

½ teaspoon ground ginger

¼ teaspoon garam masala

¼ teaspoon turmeric

¼ teaspoon ground coriander

Salt and freshly ground black pepper

Preheat a grill (or grill pan) to medium-high. Cut the eggplant crosswise into ½-inch-thick rounds and sprinkle all the pieces with kosher salt. Place the salted eggplant in a colander set in a sink and let stand for about 5 minutes.

In a small bowl, mix together the yogurt, olive oil, and remaining spices, seasoning to taste with salt and pepper.

Rinse the eggplant rounds and pat them dry. Coat them with the yogurt mixture.

Lightly oil the grill rack and grill the eggplant rounds until tender and cooked through, about 4 minutes per side, moving the rounds only to flip them.

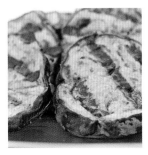

NOTE Eggplant, particularly the deep-purple-skinned variety that most of us know, has a spongy and light texture that's great for grilling. The skin is full of antioxidants and fiber. It's a very versatile vegetable and often can be used in place of meat.

NUTRITION INFORMATION: SERVING SIZE: 4–5 rounds • CALORIES: 70 • CALORIES FROM FAT: 25 • TOTAL FAT: 2.5 grams • SATURATED FAT: 0 grams • CHOLESTEROL: 0 milligrams • SODIUM: 15 milligrams • TOTAL CARBOHYDRATE: 10 grams • FIBER: 5 grams • PROTEIN: 4 grams

Pan-Fried Tofu Nuggets
with Oven-Burst Tomatoes and Broccoli

Don't be intimidated by the number of spices listed for the tofu. Yes, it's a lot, but the broccoli and tomato are so minimally spiced that the overall effect is very balanced. Although it's tempting to shake the pan while the tofu nuggets cook, try to keep it to a minimum so that the tofu gets crispy on the outside.

Serves 4

25 cherry tomatoes, preferably a mix of colors

Olive oil, for spraying

½ head of broccoli, cut into large florets

1 lemon, halved

1 teaspoon garlic powder

1 teaspoon paprika

1 teaspoon ground cumin

⅛ teaspoon cayenne

1 tablespoon dried thyme

1 tablespoon sesame seeds

Salt and pepper

1 package firm tofu, cut into 1-inch cubes

2 tablespoons olive oil

Preheat the oven to 400°F. Spread the tomatoes on a baking sheet, spray lightly with olive oil, and roast until the tomatoes begin to burst, about 15 minutes. Transfer the tomatoes to a plate and increase the heat to 450°F. Arrange the broccoli on the baking sheet, spray lightly with oil, and roast until just brown around the edges, about 10 minutes. Remove from the oven and squeeze the lemon juice over the broccoli.

In a large bowl, whisk together the garlic powder, paprika, cumin, cayenne, thyme, and sesame seeds; season to taste with salt and pepper. Add the cubes of tofu and toss until coated.

Heat the olive oil in a large pan over medium-high heat. Add the tofu and cook, turning only occasionally, until browned, 6–7 minutes. Remove from the heat and gently toss together the tofu, broccoli, and tomatoes, taking care not to lose all the juices from the tomatoes.

NOTE Tofu, made from soybeans, often is considered tasteless or boring. Although it's true that tofu isn't for everyone, when it's prepared well, it's quite delicious. It truly will take on the flavors of other ingredients, and so a good tofu recipe depends on preparation and complementary ingredients.

NUTRITION INFORMATION: SERVING SIZE: about 1 cup • **CALORIES:** 190 • **CALORIES FROM FAT:** 110 • **TOTAL FAT:** 12 grams • **SATURATED FAT:** 1.5 grams • **CHOLESTEROL:** 0 milligrams • **SODIUM:** 55 milligrams • **TOTAL CARBOHYDRATE:** 12 grams • **FIBER:** 4 grams • **PROTEIN:** 12 grams

Lemony
Spaghetti Squash

A common recommendation when trying to cut carbs is to substitute spaghetti squash for actual spaghetti. Although most of those "pastas" focus on tomato sauces, I think spaghetti squash pasta is perfect for the time between winter and spring, when winter squash is still available and spring peas are just coming into season. However, here I've made it with frozen peas to ensure the sweetness critical to the classic lemon-pea-Parmesan combination.

Serves 4

1 spaghetti squash, halved and seeded

1 tablespoon olive oil

2 cloves garlic, minced

1½ cups frozen peas, defrosted

3 tablespoons chopped fresh parsley leaves

3 sprigs chopped oregano

Finely grated zest and juice of 1 lemon

½ cup grated Parmesan cheese

Salt and freshly ground black pepper

Preheat the oven to 350°. Fill a roasting pan with about 1 inch of water and place the spaghetti squash in it, cut side down. Roast until it is easily pierced with a fork, 20–25 minutes. When it is cool enough to handle, use a fork to scrape the sides of the squash to form strands until all of the flesh is removed; you should have about 3 cups. Drain the squash in a colander.

Meanwhile, heat the oil in a large pan over medium heat. Add the garlic and cook, stirring occasionally, until softened and fragrant, 2–3 minutes. Turn the heat down to low and add the peas, parsley, and oregano. Toss well and heat just until the peas are heated through; do not cook them. Remove from the heat and toss together the pea mixture, squash, lemon zest and juice, and Parmesan; season to taste with salt and pepper.

NOTE One cup of spaghetti (which is more than double a serving size but typical of many restaurant portions) has more than 400 calories and 40 grams of carbohydrates. Spaghetti squash, in contrast, has about 40 calories and less than 10 grams of carbohydrate in 1 cup. It also has more vitamins (such as vitamin A) and minerals (such as potassium) and is in general a healthier choice. Though the texture is a little different, spaghetti squash is a great low-carb addition to meals.

NUTRITION INFORMATION: SERVING SIZE: ¾ cup • CALORIES: 120 • CALORIES FROM FAT: 50 • TOTAL FAT: 5 grams • SATURATED FAT: 2 grams • CHOLESTEROL: 10 milligrams • SODIUM: 180 milligrams • TOTAL CARBOHYDRATE: 13 grams • FIBER: 4 grams • PROTEIN: 6 grams

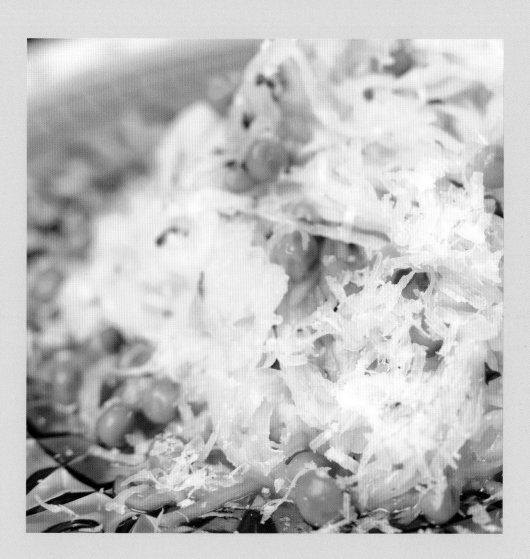

Spicy
Kale Chips

There are a lot of kale chip recipes online that suggest different cooking times and temperatures. After testing a lot of them, I feel confident reporting that this recipe pinpoints the making of a great chip. In my opinion, preparing only one bunch of kale is never enough.

Serves 4

8 cups chopped kale or 1 bunch torn into ½- to 1-inch pieces

1 tablespoon olive oil

1 teaspoon paprika

1 teaspoon ground cumin

Pinch of cayenne

Salt and freshly ground black pepper

Preheat the oven to 300°F. Line a baking sheet with parchment paper.

Dry the kale as thoroughly as possible and put it in a large bowl. Add the olive oil, paprika, cumin, and cayenne, and toss well; season to taste with salt and pepper.

Arrange the kale in a single layer on the baking sheet. Bake, turning once or twice, until crisp, about 20 minutes. Let cool slightly before eating.

NOTE We all know kale is healthy from its recent 15 minutes of fame, but just how healthy is it? Ounce for ounce, it has more vitamin C than an orange, more vitamins A and K than any other leafy green, and more calcium than milk.

NUTRITION INFORMATION: SERVING SIZE: ½ cup • CALORIES: 100 • CALORIES FROM FAT: 40 • TOTAL FAT: 4.5 grams • SATURATED FAT: 0.5 gram • CHOLESTEROL: 0 milligrams • SODIUM: 60 milligrams • TOTAL CARBOHYDRATE: 14 grams • FIBER: 3 grams • PROTEIN: 5 grams

Pecan Pumpkin Tamales

For years my family celebrated Thanksgiving at my great-aunt's beautiful old, creaky house, but when she decided she was no longer up to the challenge of hosting 30 people for the holiday, my mom and I had the honor of inheriting the family tradition. But we are not traditional. (We like to think of it as breathing new life into one of our favorite holidays.) The first year we hosted, I had recently begun working as a nutrition educator and cooking demonstrator in New York City and had just tasted my first real tamales. When we ventured into the world of tamale making, we knew we couldn't match the expertise of long-standing family recipes and techniques, and so we decided to go our own, American way.

Makes 10 tamales

About 15 dried corn husks

⅓ cup chopped pecans

1¼ cups corn flour (masa harina)

1¼ cup pumpkin puree

⅓ cup low-sodium chicken broth

¼ cup unsalted butter, melted

1 teaspoon cinnamon

½ teaspoon allspice

½ teaspoon freshly grated nutmeg

½ teaspoon ground ginger

¼ teaspoon ground cloves

¼ teaspoon salt

In a large bowl, clean and separate the corn husks. Soak them in warm water for at least 30 minutes to soften. Then toast the pecans in a small pan over medium-low heat until fragrant, 4–5 minutes. Remove from the heat.

In a large bowl, combine the corn flour, pumpkin puree, chicken broth, butter, reserved pecans, and spices and stir well.

Tear 5 of the soaked corn husks into strips, which you will use to hold the tamales closed. Spoon about 3 tablespoons of the corn flour mixture onto a corn husk. Fold the sides inward and roll the husk closed. Tie a piece of husk around the tamale to keep it closed. Repeat with the remaining husks and masa mixture.

Bring a large pot of water fitted with a strainer to a boil. Place the tamales inside and steam until tender and cooked through, about 45 minutes.

NOTE True tamales are made with lard and masa harina, and so the texture is vastly different from the tamales in this recipe. But the tamale-making technique is fantastic: an inedible husk helps keep the bundle together while preserving flavor and moisture as it steams. Plus, tamales date back thousands of years to the Mayan people and have been made with meat, fruit, fish, and vegetables. Thus, although this recipe is a vegetable-centric take, you can make a masa harina dough and stuff it with all types of ingredients.

NUTRITION INFORMATION: SERVING SIZE: 1 tamale • CALORIES: 130 • CALORIES FROM FAT: 70 • TOTAL FAT: 8 grams • SATURATED FAT: 3 grams • CHOLESTEROL: 10 milligrams • SODIUM: 50 milligrams • TOTAL CARBOHYDRATE: 14 grams • FIBER: 3 grams • PROTEIN: 2 grams

Escarole and Beans
with Pecorino Cheese

Though this dish sounds fairly mundane, it is modeled after the best thing I ever ate: a dish of the same name from a small Italian restaurant in the Northeast. I spent years trying to replicate that version and failed to do so until I stumbled upon the technique used here: taking the time to create a light but very flavorful chicken and garlic broth. You'll be amazed at the difference you taste with this simple change.

Serves 15

2 sprigs thyme

1 sprig rosemary

4 cups low-sodium chicken broth

3 cloves garlic, peeled

1 can pink beans, drained and rinsed

1 can black beans, drained and rinsed

1 can butter beans, drained and rinsed

1 tablespoon olive oil

2 heads escarole, roughly chopped

⅓ cup grated fresh Pecorino

Tie the thyme and rosemary sprigs together with kitchen twine. Add the herb bundle to a large pan, along with the chicken broth and garlic. Bring to a simmer over medium heat and simmer until the broth is reduced by half, about 10 minutes. Reduce the heat to low and add all the beans and the olive oil. Cook until the beans are heated through, 5–6 minutes, and then gently add the escarole, taking care not to bruise it. Cook until the escarole has softened but remains bright green, about 5 minutes. Remove from the heat. To serve, ladle ½ cup portions into bowls and sprinkle with Pecorino cheese.

NOTE Escarole is not a wildly popular leafy green because it's not packed full of nutrients in the same way that kale or spinach is, but it's unique because it can be both light and hearty. During cooking, it doesn't break down as quickly as lettuce does, but the light flavor and texture make it ideal for a delicate dish.

NUTRITION INFORMATION: SERVING SIZE: ½ cup • CALORIES: 110 • CALORIES FROM FAT: 20 • TOTAL FAT: 2 grams • SATURATED FAT: 0.5 gram • CHOLESTEROL: 0 milligrams • SODIUM: 240 milligrams • TOTAL CARBOHYDRATE: 17 grams • FIBER: 5 grams • PROTEIN: 7 grams

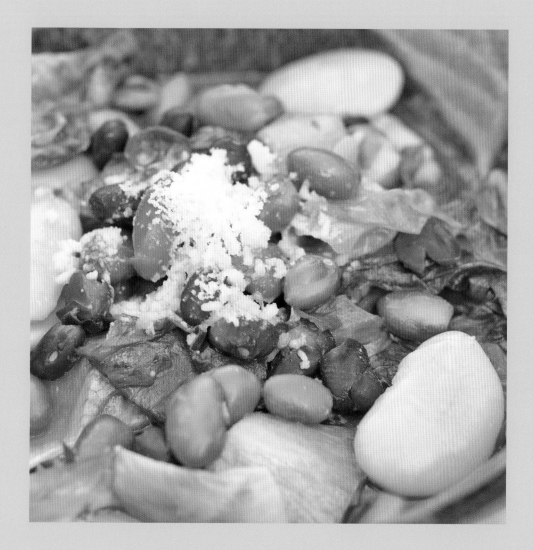

Desserts

Dessert doesn't have to be a dirty word in a diabetic person's mealtime lexicon—treats are a necessary component to satisfy a sweet tooth. The key to dessert is simply portion sizing, which is why many of the recipes in this section—treats like Mini Chocolate Orange Cakes with Ancho Chilies and Coconut Chia Seed and Lemon Pudding—are prepared in individual servings. I've created luscious desserts without overloading on sugar—a happy end to a whole (food) meal.

Chewy Almond Cookies
with Cherry Bourbon Preserves

These cookies are very much like French macaroons but have much less sugar. Changing the sugar content alters the texture of the cookie—in my opinion, it's no better or worse, just different. The almond extract really makes these cookies pop.

Serves 6

Cookies

2 egg whites

1 teaspoon almond extract

Pinch of salt

½ cup powdered sugar

½ cup almond flour

Sauce

1 cup pitted fresh or frozen cherries

2 tablespoons bourbon

Preheat the oven to 300°F. Beat together the egg whites, almond extract, and salt until soft peaks form. Gradually add in the powdered sugar, beating constantly, until the egg whites become glossy and form stiff peaks (the egg whites stand up when the beaters are drawn out). Gently fold in the almond flour.

Place the mixture in a plastic bag and cut off one of the corners to make a pastry bag. Pipe out 12 cookies, about 1 inch each, onto a baking sheet lined with parchment paper. Let the cookies dry for 10–15 minutes in a cool place.

Bake the cookies for about 15 minutes, rotating the pan halfway though and leaving the the oven door propped open slightly (using a wooden spoon) for the last 2–3 minutes of baking or until the edges of the cookies turn golden. When finished, slide the parchment paper onto a cooking rack.

While the cookies bake, bring the cherries and bourbon to a boil in a small saucepan. After the cherries have softened, use a potato masher to gently break apart the fruit. Continue to boil until thickened and reduced, 7–8 minutes. Remove from the heat and let cool.

To serve, spread a little of the preserves on each cookie.

NOTE Cookies, which are usually very high in carbohydrates because of the sugar and flour, don't have to be. Because of their use of egg whites and almond flour, French macaroons are a step in the right direction. However, traditional macaroons have a lot of sugar and often have a rich, sugary filling, so take care.

NUTRITION INFORMATION: SERVING SIZE: 2 cookies • CALORIES: 120 • CALORIES FROM FAT: 40 • TOTAL FAT: 4.5 grams • SATURATED FAT: 0 grams • CHOLESTEROL: 0 milligrams • SODIUM: 20 milligrams • TOTAL CARBOHYDRATE: 16 grams • FIBER: 2 grams • PROTEIN: 3 grams

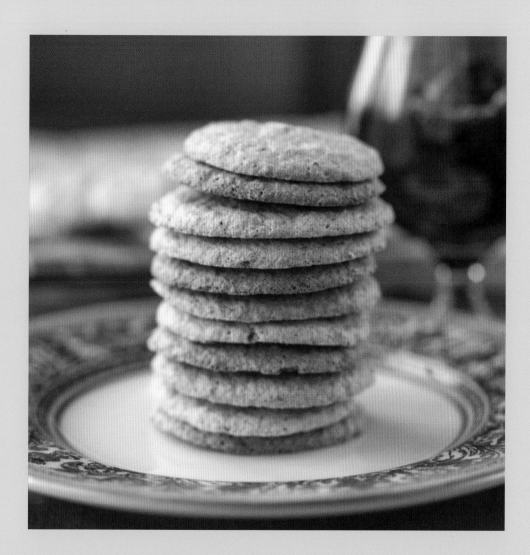

Mini Chocolate Orange Cakes
with Ancho Chilies

The chili-orange-chocolate combo is a cross-cultural favorite. When I set out to develop a chocolate cake recipe for this book, I knew I didn't want it to be overly sweet, because no artificial sweeteners are needed to make delicious and healthy desserts.

Makes: 18

2 cups almond flour (or 6–7 ounces of whole almonds, finely ground using a food processor or blender)

¾ cup sugar, divided

5 ounces cacao beans, finely ground

1 tablespoon ancho chili powder

6 large eggs, separated

1 teaspoon vanilla extract

½ cup unsweetened cocoa powder

1 cup freshly squeezed orange juice (from 2 large oranges)

3 teaspoons finely grated orange zest

¼ teaspoon salt

1 cup whipping cream

Preheat oven to 350°F. Lightly spray muffin tins (enough to hold 18 cups) with olive or vegetable oil. Combine almond flour, ¼ cup sugar, ground cacao, and ancho chili powder in a medium-size bowl.

In a large bowl, combine the egg yolks, vanilla, and ¼ cup sugar. Beat or whisk the mixture until it is thick and creamy. Whisk in the cocoa powder, orange juice, and orange zest. Fold in the almond flour mixture.

In a separate bowl, beat the egg whites and salt together until soft peaks form. While beating constantly, slowly add 3 tablespoons sugar, scraping down the sides as needed. Beat until glossy, stiff peaks form, 3–4 minutes. Gently fold the egg white mixture into the batter, folding until just barely incorporated; do not overmix. Divide the batter evenly among the 18 cups and bake until a toothpick inserted into the middle comes out clean, about 20 minutes. Let cool.

Whip the cream and the remaining 1 tablespoon sugar until fluffy. Place in a pastry bag or plastic bag and cut the corner. Pipe a little whipped cream onto each of the cupcakes.

NOTE Cacao beans are the basis of chocolate; in a sense, they are the most pure version of chocolate commercially available. When chocolate is made from cacao (which can be done at home), sugar is added, so by using the beans, you can avoid added sugar but still get the benefit of the chocolaty flavor. You'll also get the health benefits of chocolate: lots of antioxidants and heart benefits.

NUTRITION INFORMATION: SERVING SIZE: 1 minicake, plus 1 tablespoon whipped cream • CALORIES: 180 • CALORIES FROM FAT: 100 • TOTAL FAT: 11 grams • SATURATED FAT: 1 gram • CHOLESTEROL: 60 grams • SODIUM: 60 grams • TOTAL CARBOHYDRATE: 17 grams • FIBER: 2 grams • PROTEIN: 6 grams

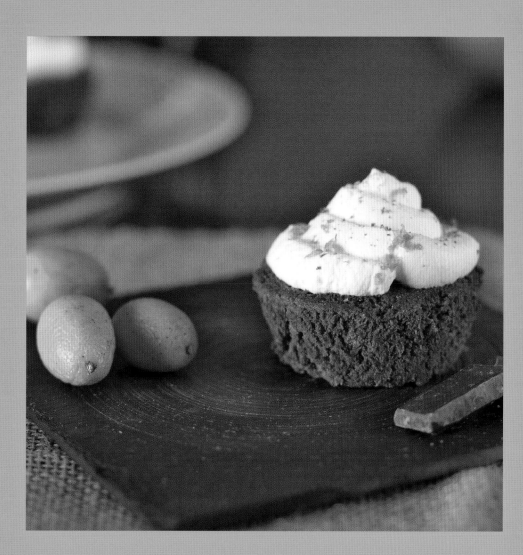

Rhubarb and Yogurt Parfait
with Flaxseed Crumble

Rhubarb has such a short season that it should be savored and preserved, mainly by making extra sauce and freezing it. By doubling or tripling the rhubarb sauce, you can make this a year-round treat.

Serves 6

3 cups chopped rhubarb

3 cups halved strawberries

2 tablespoons honey

1½ tablespoons minced crystallized ginger

1 cinnamon stick

Finely grated zest and juice of 1 lime (at least 2 tablespoons juice)

⅓ cup walnut halves

¼ cup flaxseeds

1 teaspoon ground cinnamon

2 cups plain nonfat Greek yogurt

1 teaspoon cinnamon extract

1 teaspoon vanilla extract

Combine the rhubarb, strawberries, honey, ginger, and cinnamon stick in a medium-size saucepan and bring the mixture to a boil over medium heat. Remove the cinnamon stick, add the lime juice and zest, and simmer until the mixture begins to thicken, 15–20 minutes. Using a large wooden spoon, mash any large pieces of the fruit. Remove from the heat and let cool.

Meanwhile, combine the walnuts, flaxseed, and ground cinnamon in a food processor and pulse until crumbly.

Stir together the Greek yogurt and the cinnamon and vanilla extracts in a small bowl. To serve, layer the yogurt, rhubarb, and flax seed crumble in dessert bowls or champagne glasses.

NOTE Rhubarb is one of the first spring fruits—though I use the term "fruit" loosely because rhubarb (unlike other fruits) is very tart. Plus, the leaves are poisonous. Rhubarb has been used as a medicinal treatment for a variety of conditions, including to aid digestion. It's also used as an astringent for cuts and burns.

NUTRITION INFORMATION: SERVING SIZE: 1 parfait • CALORIES: 170 • CALORIES FROM FAT: 50 • TOTAL FAT: 6 grams • SATURATED FAT: 0.5 gram • CHOLESTEROL: 0 milligrams • SODIUM: 30 milligrams • TOTAL CARBOHYDRATE: 21 grams • FIBER: 5 grams • PROTEIN: 10 grams

Baklava Bundles

Rugelach and baklava: two delicious yet high-sugar desserts. Baklava is made with nuts and honey layered between sheets of phyllo dough, and rugelach features a rich dough spread with a jammy filling and rolled up. Here the two meet to produce a dessert that's lower in carbohydrate and fat. These bundles are the perfect two-bite treat: sweet, fruity, nutty, and very filling.

Serves 12

1 large apple, cored and chopped

3 dried apricots

2 dried figs

2 dried dates

3 tablespoons chopped walnuts

2 tablespoons raisins

Juice from 1 small orange

½ teaspoon cinnamon

8 sheets phyllo dough

Olive oil sprayer

4 teaspoons sugar

1 egg

2 tablespoons water

Preheat the oven to 350°F. Spray a baking sheet lightly with oil.

In a food processor, combine the apple, apricots, figs, dates, walnuts, raisins, orange juice, and cinnamon. Pulse until combined, scraping down the sides as needed.

On a clean, dry cutting board, lay 1 phyllo sheet. Spray lightly with olive oil and sprinkle with ½ teaspoon of sugar. Lay another sheet of phyllo on top, spray with olive oil, and sprinkle with sugar; continue until you have used four sheets of phyllo. Spoon half of the fruit mixture along the long edge of the phyllo sheets closest to you and spread halfway up the sheet (away from you). Roll the phyllo and filling into a log. Slice the log crosswise in 1-inch pieces and arrange on the baking sheet. Repeat this process with the remaining phyllo sheets and filling.

In a small bowl, beat together the egg and water. Lightly brush the tops of the pastries with the egg wash and bake until golden, 30–35 minutes.

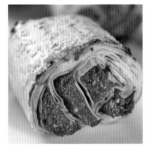

NOTE Figs and dates, like other dried fruit, tend to be very high in sugar because they're so low in water. However, in the drying process, the fruits retain most of their nutrients, and so dried fruit can be a part of healthy meals. Figs are particularly high in fiber and vitamin B_6.

NUTRITION INFORMATION: SERVING SIZE: 2 pieces • CALORIES: 90 • CALORIES FROM FAT: 30 • TOTAL FAT: 3.5 grams • SATURATED FAT: 0.5 gram • CHOLESTEROL: 15 milligrams • SODIUM: 70 milligrams • TOTAL CARBOHYDRATE: 13 grams • FIBER: 1 gram • PROTEIN: 2 grams

French Toast Quiche
with Strawberries and Basil

The sweetness of many American breakfasts makes them a perfect candidate for dessert. This sophisticated version of French toast is perfectly portioned as a satisfying but light dessert.

Serves 4

1 cup torn challah or egg dinner roll

5 egg whites

3 egg yolks

¼ cup almond milk

¼ cup brown sugar

1 teaspoon cinnamon

½ teaspoon vanilla extract

8 strawberries, finely chopped

6 fresh basil leaves, finely chopped

Preheat the oven to 325°F. Lightly spray four 6-ounce ramekins with oil, to prevent sticking. Tear the challah roll into bite-size pieces and divide aming the four ramekins. Lightly beat together the egg whites, egg yolks, almond milk, brown sugar, cinnamon, and vanilla until combined. Add about three-quarters of the chopped strawberries and about half the basil to the egg mixture and then pour the mixture evenly over the ramekins of challah.

Bake until set, 30–35 minutes. Before serving, top with the remaining chopped strawberries and basil.

NOTE Basil is a fantastically unique herb because it comes in a variety of flavors and is used differently around the world. Some varieties are spicy and hot (such as Spicy Bush and Sweet Thai basil) and are used in savory dishes such as traditional Thai foods. Other savory dishes use a cinnamon variety native to Mexico. Lemon basil, in contrast, is more mild and perfect for salads. This is only a very short list; there are more than 10 commonly consumed varieties—try experimenting with all of them.

NUTRITION INFORMATION: SERVING SIZE: 1 (6-ounce) ramekin • CALORIES: 120 • CALORIES FROM FAT: 35 • TOTAL FAT: 4 grams • SATURATED FAT: 1.5 grams • CHOLESTEROL: 140 milligrams • SODIUM: 120 milligrams • TOTAL CARBOHYDRATE: 13 grams • FIBER: 0 grams • PROTEIN: 7 grams

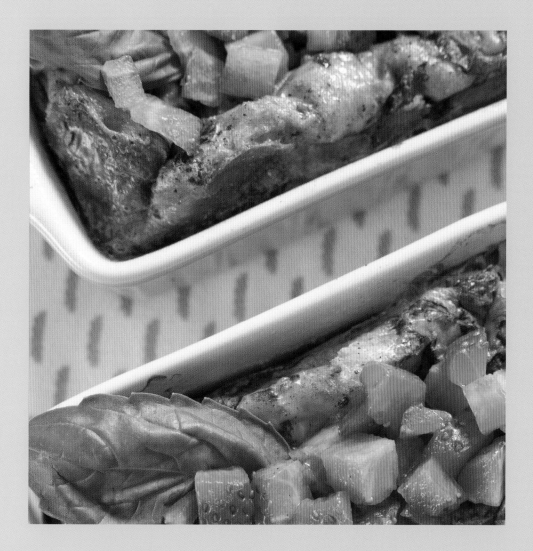

Maple Almond
Panna Cotta

Creamy desserts often come with a costly and caloric price: extra fat and extra sugar. If you use Greek yogurt, a thick and high-protein alternative to cream, you get the same consistency in a healthier way.

Serves 4

1½ teaspoons unflavored powdered gelatin

1 tablespoon cold water

1 cup almond milk

2 tablespoons maple syrup

1 cup 2 percent Greek yogurt

1 cup buttermilk

1½ teaspoons almond extract

¼ cup slivered almonds

1 cup halved blueberries

Mix together the gelatin and water in a small bowl and let stand 5 minutes to soften.

Bring the almond milk to a simmer in a small saucepan over low heat and then stir in the maple syrup and cook for about 1 minute. Remove from the heat. Add the gelatin, stirring, until dissolved.

Whisk together the yogurt, buttermilk, and almond extract until very smooth. Whisk in the warm milk until smooth. Pour the mixture into four ramekins and refrigerate until set, about 3 hours.

To serve, top the panna cottas (in the ramekins) with the slivered almonds and blueberries.

Note: When selecting almond milk, choose one without added ingredients. Usually processors add "stabilizers" so that the milk doesn't separate, but they're not really necessary. If none of the supermarket options are to your liking, don't be afraid to make your own.

NOTE Panna cotta is Italian for "cooked cream." "Cream" generally signifies a high-sugar, high-fat dessert, but less decadent, equally delicious versions can be made. Almond milk is underused in desserts; it provides depth and flavor without adding sugar.

NUTRITION INFORMATION: SERVING SIZE: ½ cup • CALORIES: 150 • CALORIES FROM FAT: 45 • TOTAL FAT: 5 grams • SATURATED FAT: 1.5 grams • CHOLESTEROL: 5 milligrams • SODIUM: 125 milligrams • TOTAL CARBOHYDRATE: 16 grams • FIBER: 1 gram • PROTEIN: 9 grams

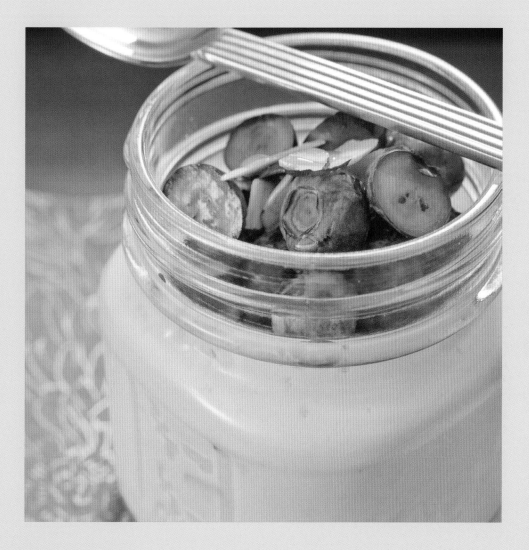

How to Make Almond Milk in 5 Easy Steps

1. Prepare the almonds. Soak raw almonds (covered) overnight or up to two days. The longer the nuts soak, the creamier the milk. Drain and rinse the almonds.

2. Add almonds and water to a blender or food processor in a 1:2 ratio (1 cup of almonds with 2 cups of water). Blend for 2–4 minutes (longer in food processors). The nuts should be a very fine meal with a white, opaque milk when you're done.

3. Strain the almond mixture: Line a fine-mesh strainer with cheesecloth and place over a bowl. When most of the liquid has drained, wrap the cheesecloth around the almond meal, twist, and squeeze to extract as much of the milk as possible.

4. Sweeten if needed. (I like to use a little bit of maple syrup or wildflower honey.)

5. Enjoy! The milk can be used for two days. The almond meal can be dried and added to oatmeal or baked goods or frozen for up to 6 months.

Pumpkin Pie Pockets

One of the challenges of pie is that no matter how delicious (or low in sugar) the filling is, the crust is still packed with fat and carbohydrates. This is why I recommend getting rid of it altogether! Use phyllo dough instead, which can be made healthier by using only a little oil between sheets and only a few sheets per pie pocket.

Serves 10

1½ cups canned pumpkin puree

½ cup 2 percent plain Greek yogurt

½ cup 2 percent milk

½ cup packed brown sugar

3 large eggs plus 2 large egg yolks, lightly beaten

2 tablespoons minced crystallized ginger

1 teaspoon ground cinnamon

½ teaspoon freshly ground nutmeg

½ teaspoon salt

¼ teaspoon ground cloves

10 sheets phyllo dough

Olive oil sprayer

Preheat the oven to 350°F. Place the pumpkin puree, yogurt, milk, brown sugar, eggs, egg yolks, crystallized ginger, cinnamon, nutmeg, salt, and cloves in a blender. Blend until combined and smooth. Pour the mixture into a 9 × 13–inch baking dish. Bake until a toothpick inserted in the center comes out clean, about 45 minutes. Let cool (keep the oven on).

Lay 1 sheet of phyllo on a clean, dry cutting board. Spray lightly with olive oil and top with another phyllo sheet. Cut the phyllo stack lengthwise into four strips. Scoop out 2 tablespoons of the pumpkin pie mixture and place it on the bottom corner of one of the phyllo strips. Fold the corner of the phyllo over to enclose the filling, forming a triangle. Continue folding the strip (like a flag), maintaining the triangle shape, until you reach the end of the phyllo strip. Repeat with the remaining pieces of phyllo and pumpkin pie mixture (you should have 20 pie pockets).

Spray a baking sheet lightly with oil and arrange the pie pockets on it in a single layer. Spray the tops with oil and bake until golden, 15–20 minutes.

NOTE Phyllo dough is a healthier alternative to puff pastry or regular pastry crust. This extremely thin dough is used on a per-sheet basis and can be used in smaller amounts, whereas the layers of puff pastry can't be separated. Thus, puff pastry also has a lot more fat.

NUTRITION INFORMATION: SERVING SIZE: 2 pockets • CALORIES: 160 • CALORIES FROM FAT: 45 • TOTAL FAT: 5 grams • SATURATED FAT: 1.5 grams • CHOLESTEROL: 100 milligrams • SODIUM: 130 milligrams • TOTAL CARBOHYDRATE: 20 grams • FIBER: 1 gram • PROTEIN: 6 grams

Blueberry Lemon
Ricotta Cake

Eggs, lemon, and blueberry are a natural combination. When I first made this recipe, I was hoping to make it a breakfast bar; instead, it tasted so decadent that it made better sense as a sweet treat.

Serves 12

Egg cake
- 1 cup all-purpose flour
- ⅓ cup sugar, plus a little extra for sprinkling
- ½ teaspoon salt
- 4 large or jumbo eggs, separated
- ⅔ cup part-skim ricotta, drained in cheesecloth
- 2 tablespoons butter, melted
- Finely grated zest and juice of 1 lemon (about ⅓ cup juice)
- 1 cup fresh or frozen blueberries

Blueberry sauce
- 3 cups blueberries, fresh or frozen and thawed
- ½ cup sugar

Preheat the oven to 375°F. Place a 9 × 9–inch square baking dish in the oven to preheat while you assemble the cake.

To make the cake, combine the flour, sugar, and salt in a large bowl. In another bowl, whisk together the egg yolks, ricotta, butter, lemon juice, and lemon zest until evenly combined. Slowly add the dry ingredients to the wet ingredients, mixing as you go.

In a small bowl, whip the egg whites until stiff peaks form. Fold the whites into the batter. Gently fold in the blueberries, reserving some to sprinkle on top.

Remove the hot baking dish from the oven and spray with cooking oil. Add the batter to the dish and then sprinkle with the reserved blueberries and a little sugar. Bake until the top is slightly browned, about 20 minutes. Let cool.

To make the blueberry sauce, combine the blueberries and sugar in a saucepan over medium heat and simmer until the sugar has dissolved and the sauce begins to thicken, 5–6 minutes.

To serve, cut the cake into 12 pieces and serve each with 1½ tablespoons blueberry sauce.

NOTE Although many people think of sponge cake as an egg cake (and a delicious one), a more substantial cake can be made with eggs. A denser cake can stand up to bolder flavors and when made properly doesn't taste as though you just forgot the sugar. Many low-carb cakes turn to artificial sweeteners, but using natural ingredients to enhance the flavor is a better, healthier choice.

NUTRITION INFORMATION: SERVING SIZE: 1 square • CALORIES: 114 • CALORIES FROM FAT: 42 • TOTAL FAT: 5 grams • SATURATED FAT: 2 grams • CHOLESTEROL: 0 milligrams • SODIUM: 50 milligrams • TOTAL CARBOHYDRATE: 14 grams • FIBER: 1 gram • PROTEIN: 5 grams

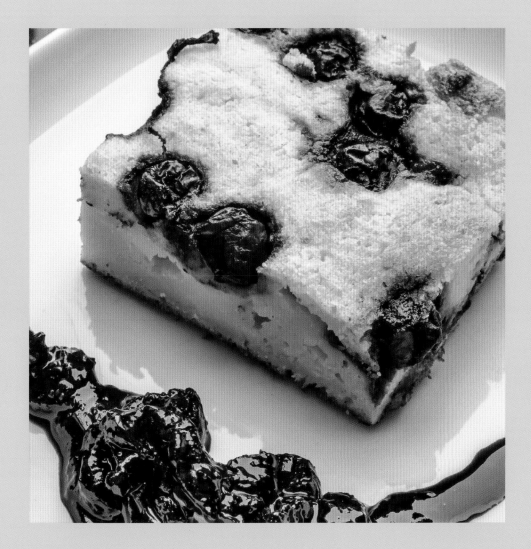

Coconut Chia Seed and
Lemon Pudding

Homemade lemon curd is a sweet and luscious dessert. Unfortunately, it is packed with fat and sugar and the protein content is basically nil. This recipe takes advantage of that sweetness but tones it down by mixing the lemon curd with Greek yogurt and adding chia seeds to the coconut milk. These small changes never fail to impress.

Serves 6

1 cup unsweetened coconut milk

¾ cup warm water

¼ cup chia seeds

½ teaspoon vanilla extract

4 egg yolks

¼ cup sugar

⅓ cup freshly squeezed lemon juice and zest

1 teaspoon unsalted butter

¾ cup plain nonfat Greek yogurt

1 pint raspberries

Combine the coconut milk, water, chia seeds, and vanilla in a medium-size bowl. Let sit for 1 hour, stirring every 15 minutes.

Meanwhile, make the lemon curd. Create a double boiler by setting a metal bowl over a pot of simmering water (make sure the bottom of the bowl does not touch the water). Whisk the egg yolks and sugar together in the bowl. Once the sugar is dissolved, whisk in the lemon juice and zest. Continue whisking until the mixture is thick enough to coat the back of a spoon, 6–7 minutes. Remove from the heat and whisk in the butter (you should have about 2 cups lemon curd). Transfer to a bowl to cool completely.

Combine the cooled lemon curd and yogurt and mix well. To assemble, spoon thin layers of the lemon curd and chia seed mixtures in small clear bowls or martini glasses. Refrigerate for 2–3 hours. Just before serving, top with the fresh raspberries.

NOTE Chia are ancient seeds that have recently become popular for their high omega-3 content. An alternative to flax, they're a little more versatile and don't need to be ground for your body to absorb the nutrients. Chia seeds gel together when mixed with a liquid, so for puddings they do all the work themselves and have a mouth feel similar to that of tapioca.

NUTRITION INFORMATION: SERVING SIZE: ⅓ cup • CALORIES: 200 • CALORIES FROM FAT: 120 • TOTAL FAT: 14 grams • SATURATED FAT: 8 grams • CHOLESTEROL: 125 milligrams • SODIUM: 25 milligrams • TOTAL CARBOHYDRATE: 17 grams • FIBER: 5 grams • PROTEIN: 7 grams

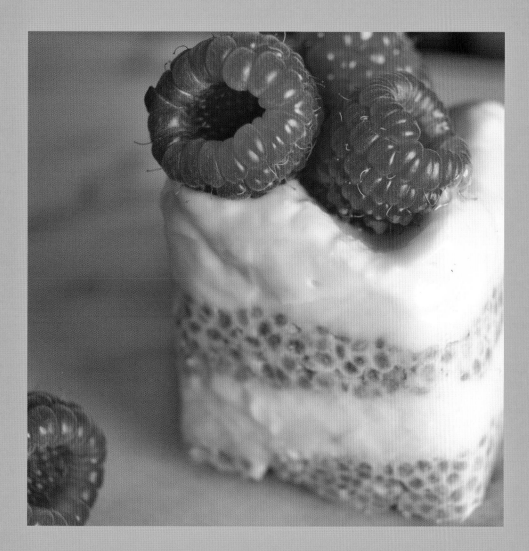

Pecan Crostini
with Blueberry Compote and Chèvre

This recipe's individual ingredients really come alive in combination. The twice-baked crostini can be made well in advance, making this a perfect single-bite party dessert.

Serves 8

Crostini
- ⅔ cup chopped pecans
- ½ cup whole-wheat pastry flour
- 2 teaspoons dried thyme
- ½ teaspoon baking soda
- ¼ teaspoon salt, plus pinch for compote
- ¼ cup nonfat, plain Greek yogurt
- ¼ cup skim milk
- 1½ tablespoons wildflower honey
- 1 cup blueberries, fresh or frozen
- 4–5 slices fresh ginger

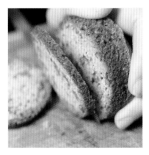

Preheat the oven to 350°F. Spray a muffin tin lightly with olive oil or cooking spray.

Toast the pecans in a medium-size pan over medium heat, stirring occasionally, until golden and fragrant, about 6–7 minutes. Transfer to a plate and set aside to cool.

Whisk together the flour, dried thyme, baking soda, and ¼ teaspoon salt in a large bowl. In another bowl, whisk together the yogurt, milk, and honey. Add the wet ingredients to the flour mixture and mix until combined. Fold in the pecans.

Fill each muffin cup about ¾ full with batter. Bake until the tops are lightly golden and a toothpick comes out clean, 15–20 minutes. Remove the muffins from the pan and let cool. When cooled completely, wrap each muffin in aluminum foil and freeze for several hours (this will make them easier to cut into rounds).

Preheat the oven to 300°F. Remove the muffins from the freezer and, using a serrated knife, slice each muffin crosswise into ⅛-inch-thick rounds (you should have about 24 rounds). Arrange the rounds in a single layer on a baking sheet and bake, flipping once halfway through, until the rounds are golden and crisp, 10–15 minutes. Transfer to a rack to cool.

Combine the blueberries, ginger, fresh thyme, and vinegar in a medium-size saucepan. Bring to a boil over medium-high heat and then reduce the heat to low and simmer for 15 minutes. Using a slotted spoon, crush some of the blueberries so that there is a mixture of crushed and whole berries. Remove the pan from the heat and season with a tiny pinch of salt. Let cool.

Once cooled, spread about ½ tablespoon of chèvre onto each crostino (this will create a barrier so that the compote doesn't soften the crostini too much) and top with a spoonful of blueberry compote.

1 tablespoon sherry
  vinegar

1 teaspoon finely
  chopped fresh thyme
  leaves

¾ cup chèvre

NOTE Pecans, like most nuts, have a lot of heart-healthy benefits: they are rich in unsaturated fats, vitamin E, and trace minerals. Specifically, pecans are known for being the nut highest in antioxidants, which may help prevent cancer, heart disease, and Alzheimer's and Parkinson's diseases.

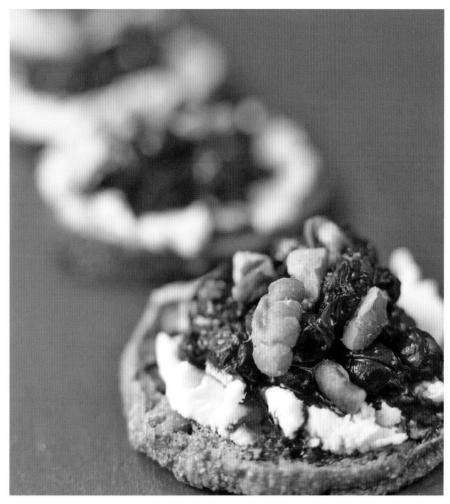

NUTRITION INFORMATION: SERVING SIZE: 3 crostini • CALORIES: 160 • CALORIES FROM FAT: 90 • TOTAL FAT: 10 grams • SATURATED FAT: 2.5 grams • CHOLESTEROL: 5 milligrams • SODIUM: 135 milligrams • TOTAL CARBOHYDRATE: 15 grams • FIBER: 3 grams • PROTEIN: 5 grams

Coconut-Ricotta Mousse
with Raspberries and Shaved Dark Chocolate

Although mousse usually isn't considered a cheesy dessert, using lightly sweetened ricotta cheese will change your perspective! Any berry will complement this dish, so use whatever is in season and available.

Serves 4

1½ cups part-skim ricotta cheese

¾ cup sweetened shredded coconut

2 tablespoons unsweetened soy milk

1 teaspoon vanilla extract

1 cup fresh raspberries

1 (1-ounce) piece 100 percent cacao dark chocolate, finely grated

Whisk together the ricotta, coconut, soy milk, and vanilla extract in a medium-size bowl until fluffy. Place a few raspberries in the bottom of four glasses (the portion size of champagne glasses works best) and then add a thin layer of grated chocolate. Top with a few tablespoons of the ricotta mixture. Continue layering with the remaining berries, chocolate, and ricotta mixture.

NOTE Ricotta is a fresh cheese that that has a slightly sweet flavor, making it ideal for desserts. It can be made easily at home with lemons and cheesecloth and is definitely worth a try. It's very versatile and will take on other flavors easily. To do so, combine 1 quart of whole milk (cow's milk is good, but sheep's milk is even better, as traditional ricotta is made with sheep's milk) and ½ cup of heavy cream in a pot and cook over medium heat until the mixture begins to boil. Turn off the heat, and add 5 tablespoons of lemon juice slowly as you stir gently. The curds will separate from the whey. Using a cheesecloth-lined sieve, drain the milk solids until the cheese reaches the desired consistency. Season to taste with salt.

NUTRITION INFORMATION: SERVING SIZE: 1 parfait • CALORIES: 200 • CALORIES FROM FAT: 110 • TOTAL FAT: 13 grams • SATURATED FAT: 9 grams • CHOLESTEROL: 30 milligrams • SODIUM: 125 milligrams • TOTAL CARBOHYDRATE: 11 gram • FIBER: 3 grams • PROTEIN: 12 grams

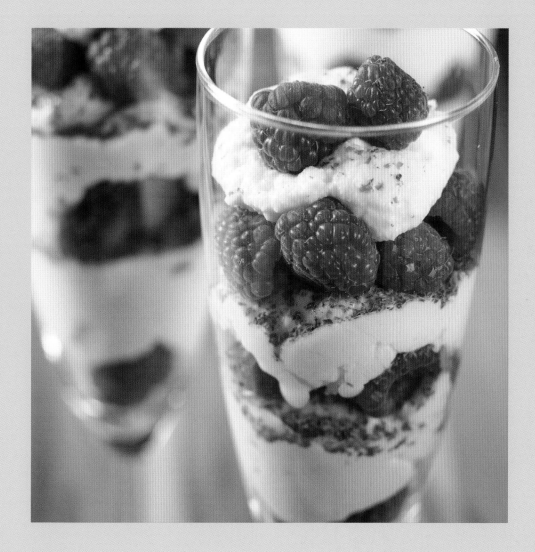

Grilled Peaches
with Minted Mascarpone

Grilling fruit brings out natural sugars that can turn slightly underripe fruits into juicy bites. Adding just a little creamy, sweet mascarpone brightens the flavor.

Serves 6

6 peaches

3 tablespoons mascarpone

½ teaspoon mint extract

½ teaspoon vanilla extract

Olive oil, for spraying

2 teaspoons fresh mint leaves, thinly sliced

Preheat a grill to medium-high. Cut the peaches in half and remove the pits. In a small bowl, stir together the mascarpone and the mint and vanilla extracts until smooth.

Spray the cut side of each peach lightly with olive oil and arrange cut side down on the grill. Grill for about 4 minutes and then carefully flip and grill for 2 minutes more. Transfer the peaches to a plate and top each half with about 1½ teaspoons of the mascarpone mixture. Garnish with the fresh mint leaves and serve warm.

NOTE Yellow peaches are known for their sweet, juicy flesh; what's less known is that white-fleshed peaches are usually sweeter and even juicier. If your fruit is not completely ripe, cook it! Poaching, stewing, or grilling will enhance its sweetness, decrease any bitterness, and soften the texture. When grilling, it's best to choose slightly underripe fruit because it holds together well during the cooking process.

NUTRITION INFORMATION: SERVING SIZE: 2 peach halves • CALORIES: 190 • CALORIES FROM FAT: 130 • TOTAL FAT: 14 grams • SATURATED FAT: 7 grams • CHOLESTEROL: 35 milligrams • SODIUM: 15 milligrams • TOTAL CARBOHYDRATE: 14 grams • FIBER: 2 grams • PROTEIN: 3 grams

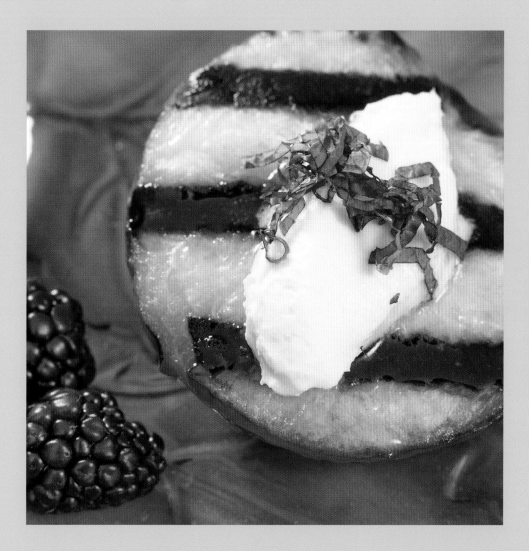

Lemon-Lavender, Pomegranate, and
Vanilla Bean Gelée

I loved Jell-O as a kid, but as I grew up, I realized that it didn't taste like much more than artificially flavored sugar. Making your own gelée is a great way to enjoy a light dessert without all the artificial flavors and sweeteners. The layering produces a nice effect, but if you're short on time, you can refrigerate the layers individually, which will produce the same flavor with less hassle.

Serves 10

Vanilla yogurt layer

- 1 tablespoon unflavored gelatin
- 2 tablespoons cold water
- 1¼ cups skim milk
- ¾ cup nonfat plain Greek yogurt
- ¼ cup sugar
- 1 sprig fresh mint
- 1 vanilla bean, split lengthwise (insides scraped, pod reserved)

Pomegranate layer

- 1 tablespoon unflavored gelatin
- ½ cup plus 2 tablespoons cold water
- 1½ cups unsweetened pomegranate juice

To make the vanilla yogurt layer, stir the gelatin into the water in a small bowl and let sit for 5 minutes to soften. Combine the milk, yogurt, sugar, and mint in a saucepan. Scrape the vanilla seeds into the mixture and add the pod. Heat over medium-low heat, stirring, until the sugar dissolves and the mixture comes to a gentle simmer. Remove from the heat. Discard the vanilla bean pod and mint sprig and stir in the gelatin until smooth. Pour the mixture into an 11 × 7–inch pan and refrigerate until set, about 1 hour.

To make the pomegranate layer, stir the gelatin into 2 tablespoons cold water in a medium-size bowl and let sit for 5 minutes to soften. Heat 1 cup pomegranate juice in a small saucepan (or in the microwave) until simmering. Remove from the heat and pour over the gelatin mixture, stirring until dissolved. Add the remaining ½ cup pomegranate juice and ½ cup cold water and stir well. Pour the mixture gently over the first layer of gelée and refrigerate 30 minutes.

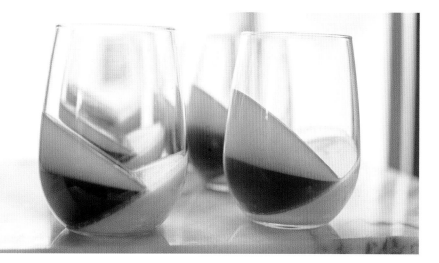

Lemon-lavender layer

- 1 tablespoon unflavored gelatin
- 1 cup plus 2 tablespoons cold water
- ¾ cup freshly squeezed lemon juice (from about 5 lemons)
- ¼ cup sugar
- 2 teaspoons dried lavender flowers

To make the lemon-lavender layer, stir the gelatin into 2 tablespoons cold water in a small bowl and let sit for 5 minutes to soften. Combine the lemon juice, sugar, and lavender flowers in a saucepan and bring to a simmer over medium heat. Line a sieve with cheesecloth and set over a medium bowl. Strain the lemon mixture, discarding the lavender, and stir in the gelatin until dissolved. Add the remaining 1 cup cold water and stir well. Pour the mixture gently over the layer of pomegranate gelée.

Refrigerate for 6 hours or overnight. Cut into 10 servings.

NOTE Lavender is an herb whose flower not only smells and tastes wonderful but has long been touted for its medicinal properties. Lavender is used to treat insomnia and aid digestion. It sometimes is used as aromatherapy to improve circulation and decrease pain (it contains oil that has a relaxing, sedative effect). There is no recommendation for how much someone should consume to get these benefits, but it can be used frequently in teas as well as in foods.

NUTRITION INFORMATION: SERVING SIZE: 1 square • CALORIES: 80 • CALORIES FROM FAT: 0 • TOTAL FAT: 0 grams • SATURATED FAT: 0 grams • CHOLESTEROL: 0 milligrams • SODIUM: 30 milligrams • TOTAL CARBOHYDRATE: 16 grams • FIBER: 0 grams • PROTEIN: 5 grams

Citrus Gratin
with Toasted Almonds

Broiling brings out the natural flavors and sweetness in fruits and is a great way to create a quick and beautiful dessert. The combination of citrus flavors in this dish makes a subtle but interesting difference and is a great way to use citrus that's about to go bad.

Serves 8

2 blood oranges

2 clementines

1 pomelo

1 pink grapefruit

1 Cara Cara orange

2 tablespoons brown sugar

2 tablespoons slivered almonds

Preheat the broiler. Peel and slice all the citrus crosswise into ⅛-inch-thick slices. Gently toss the sliced citrus with the brown sugar, rubbing in the sugar so that there are few clumps. Layer the citrus in a ceramic baking dish, sprinkle with almonds, and broil until the tops are lightly caramelized, about 8 minutes.

NOTE Citrus, as everyone knows, is packed full of vitamin C, which helps boost the immune system. However, lemons, oranges, grapefruits, and the others also provide a lot of other benefits, such as antioxidants and insoluble fiber. To get the benefit of a variety of antioxidants, consume a variety of colored fruits.

NUTRITION INFORMATION: SERVING SIZE: ½ cup slices • CALORIES: 90 • CALORIES FROM FAT: 15 • TOTAL FAT: 2 grams • SATURATED FAT: 0 grams • CHOLESTEROL: 0 milligrams • SODIUM: 50 milligrams • TOTAL CARBOHYDRATE: 16 grams • FIBER: 2 grams • PROTEIN: 2 grams

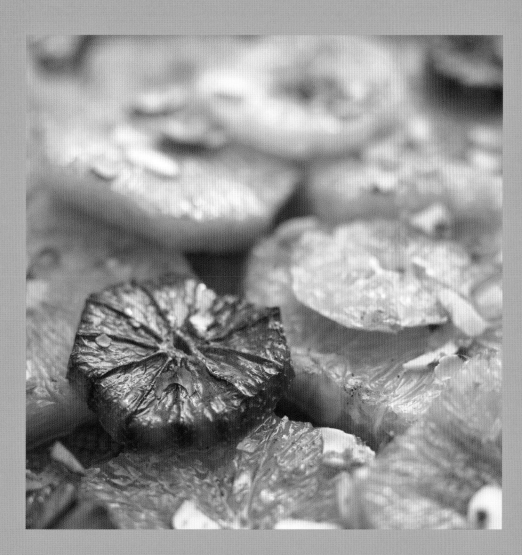

Avocado Ice Cream
with Blackberries and Shaved Dark Chocolate

When I first heard about avocado ice cream, I was skeptical. Don't get me wrong—I love fruit-based ice creams, but the savory nature of avocado didn't seem to fit. But the instant I tasted this unbelievably creamy concoction, I knew I was wrong. And you don't even need an ice cream maker—just a freezer and some willpower!

Serves 6

¼ cup skim milk

¼ cup sugar

Pinch of salt

3 ripe avocados, pitted, peeled, and roughly chopped

1 cup 2 percent plain Greek yogurt

1 teaspoon vanilla extract

1 pint blackberries

1 ounce dark chocolate, finely grated

Heat the milk, sugar, and salt in a small saucepan over low heat, stirring, until the sugar dissolves. Remove from the heat and transfer to a medium-size metal bowl, along with the avocados, yogurt, and vanilla. Using a hand blender, puree until very smooth.

Fill a larger bowl with ice. Fit the smaller bowl into the ice in the large bowl. Using a hand mixer, beat the avocado mixture until it begins to freeze, 10–15 minutes. Place the bowl of ice cream in the freezer for about 30 minutes. Remove the bowl and beat with the hand mixer again (about 5 minutes). Repeat the process one more time until the mixture is the consistency of soft-serve ice cream. Freeze the mixture for 2 more hours to firm up before serving.

Serve ½ cup of ice cream topped with blackberries and chocolate in a bowl.

Note: This recipe also can be made with a food processor or without any appliances at all. To do this, place the mixture in a resealable plastic bag and freeze it for about 4 hours, taking it out every 30 minutes and massaging the bag for about a minute each time to break up ice crystals and smooth the ice cream.

NOTE Avocados are popularly known to have healthy fats and will help the absorption of other vitamins when eaten with a salad or another vitamin-rich dish. Avocados themselves are also high in fiber, vitamin K, and folate. If you want them to ripen quickly, place them in a brown paper bag with a banana or an apple and store at room temperature; the gas the other fruit produces will help ripen the avocados quickly.

NUTRITION INFORMATION: SERVING SIZE: ½ cup • CALORIES: 210 • CALORIES FROM FAT: 140 • TOTAL FAT: 15 grams • SATURATED FAT: 2.5 grams • CHOLESTEROL: 5 milligrams • SODIUM: 25 milligrams • TOTAL CARBOHYDRATE: 17 grams • FIBER: 7 grams • PROTEIN: 6 grams

5 Kitchen Gadgets Worth Their Weight

1. **Coffee grinder**—This gadget grinds not only coffee but also spices, herbs, grains, flax seeds, other seeds, nuts, and crackers and cookies (for crusts). Be sure to purchase one that's easy to take apart and clean!

2. **Toaster oven**—Toaster ovens are incredibly versatile. In addition to toasting breads or tortillas, they bake cookies, casseroles, and meats. They melt the cheese on top of French onion soup, which is a texture and taste treat. Another plus: if you have an electric oven and use it a lot, you may be able to save a lot of money on your energy bill just by switching to a toaster oven.

3. **Panini press**—If you're going to get a panini press, make sure that it's one that has a floating hinge and can lie flat when open, which provides two additional cooking surfaces. Many panini presses come with a flat griddle and a grill pan so you can cook everything from pressing wraps to grilling vegetables or burgers.

4. **Slow cooker**—Slow cookers simplify your life when you have a lot of things to do in addition to cooking. It's very hard to overcook foods in a slow cooker, and it makes very easy, one-pot meals. Most slow cookers have multiple settings, and some even come with a stirrer mounted to the lid!

5. **Mandoline**—If you don't have a food processor, mandolines make novice cooks look like pros. They can help easily (and thinly) slice, shred, or dice fruits and vegetables. When you want to reduce your food preparation time, a mandoline is a very easy way to do it!

5 Ways to Add Flavor, not Carbs!

1. **Liquid smoke**—This flavor is exactly what it sounds like: the taste of smoke captured in water. To make liquid smoke, wood is burned, which produces tiny smoke particles in water vapor. When the vapor cools, it turns to a liquid, which is then aged in oak barrels (as wine is) to deepen the flavor.

   Use: If you want any dish you're making to taste smoky, add only a few drops of liquid smoke.

2. **Rosewater**—Extracted from roses, rosewater is used often in ethnic cuisines (particularly in desserts and drinks) of the Middle East, India, and North Africa. It adds a very nice, floral flavor.

   Use: Add it to iced tea or lemonade in place of sugar for a more floral flavor (or use it in place of vanilla extract).

3. **Flavored vinegar**—Vinegars are extremely versatile, and a little goes a long way! They are available in many different flavors that can really make a dish stand out. Currently in my kitchen are the typical three vinegars found in the home (balsamic, apple cider, and rice wine) as well as chocolate balsamic vinegar, fig balsamic vinegar, and 12-year aged white balsamic vinegar.

   Use: Add or replace vinegar with a flavored vinegar tailored to the other ingredients in the dish. For instance, I could try the chocolate vinegar with the French Toast Quiche on page 164.

4. **Saffron**—An expensive spice, saffron should be used sparingly, but it's worth the splurge! It's expensive because only three threads can be harvested from each saffron flower—and 1 ounce equals about 14,000 threads. Good-quality Spanish saffron will have a very deep red color to it.

   Tip: Don't bother wasting your money on yellowish-looking saffron or on the saffron powder, as it's often cut with something else, such as turmeric.

   Use: Add a pinch of saffron per 4–6 servings of a dish. Also, don't use wooden utensils when cooking with saffron, as wood can absorb the color and flavor of the spice.

5. **Anchovy paste**—Anchovies aren't my favorite fish, but anchovy paste is delicious! Not convinced? Have you ever had a really good Caesar salad? A key ingredient in homemade Caesar dressing is anchovies. Anchovy paste is a salty misture of ground anchovies, vinegar, oil, and sugar. It's fishy and strong, so a little goes a long way (and the tube will last in your refrigerator for many months).

   Note: A little sugar is added to the paste, but it is not enough to warrant concern or change the carbohydrate content of your meal.

   Use: Add anchovy paste to sauces, stews, chili, spreads, or tapenades, but use only a small amount at a time.

Menu Suggestions

Three-Course Menus

MENU #1

APPETIZER
Roasted Tomatillo
and Corn Soup
(18 g)

ENTRÉE
Swordfish Kebabs
with Kiwi,
Cherry Tomatoes,
and Red Onion
(16 g)

SIDE
Sweet and Spicy
Cucumber Salad
(10 g)

DESSERT
Blueberry Lemon
Ricotta Cake
(14 g)

TOTAL GRAMS OF
CARBOHYDRATES
58

MENU #2

APPETIZER
Charred Radicchio
with Cashews and
Gorgonzola
(5 g)

ENTRÉE
Walnut-Turkey
Meatballs in
Pomodoro Sauce
(22 g)

SIDE
Summer Vegetable
Pinwheel
(11 g)

DESSERT
Baklava Bundles
(13 g)

TOTAL GRAMS OF
CARBOHYDRATES
51

MENU #3

APPETIZER
Shaved Brussels
Sprouts with a
Fried Egg and
Spiced Pine Nut
Crumble
(11 g)

ENTRÉE AND SIDE
Sautéed Branzino
with a
Beluga Lentil and
Spinach Ragout
(30 g)

DESSERT
Maple Almond
Panna Cotta
(16 g)

TOTAL GRAMS OF
CARBOHYDRATES
57

MENU #4

APPETIZER
Watermelon and
Tomato Salad with
Balsamic Reduction
(19 g)

ENTRÉE
Rosemary and Mint
Marinated Lamb Chops
(2 g)

SIDE
Whole-Grain
Mustardy Cauliflower
with Raisins and Leeks
(18 g)

DESSERT
Grilled Peaches with
Minted Mascarpone
(14 g)

TOTAL GRAMS OF
CARBOHYDRATES
53

Two-Course Menus

MENU #1

APPETIZER
Salmon Carpaccio
on Homemade
Bagel Chips
(27 g)

ENTRÉE
Pasta-Free Butternut
Squash Lasagna
(13 g)

TOTAL GRAMS OF
CARBOHYDRATES
40

MENU #2

APPETIZER
Spicy Avocado
Gazpacho
(30 g)

ENTRÉE
Whole Roasted Trout
with Fennel
and Sage
(3 g)

TOTAL GRAMS OF
CARBOHYDRATES
33

MENU #3

ENTRÉE
Coconut Crusted
Chicken in a
Curry Broth
(29 g)

SIDE
Balsamic Glazed Beets
with Garlic Scapes
(15 g)

TOTAL GRAMS OF
CARBOHYDRATES
44

MENU #4

ENTRÉE
Summer Quinoa
Casserole with
Snowpeas
(28 g)

DESSERT
Maple Almond
Panna Cotta
(16 g)

TOTAL GRAMS OF
CARBOHYDRATES
44

MENU #5

APPETIZER
Buffalo Chicken
Cigars
(16 g)

ENTRÉE
Grilled Cauliflower
Steaks with a
Nutmeg-Cayenne
"Cream" Sauce
(20 g)

TOTAL GRAMS OF
CARBOHYDRATES
36

MENU #6

ENTRÉE
Spicy Crusted
Flounder with
Plum Salsa
(23 g)

SIDE
Szechuan-Style
Green Beans
(11 g)

TOTAL GRAMS OF
CARBOHYDRATES
34

MENU #7

ENTRÉE
Stuffed Pork Tenderloin
with Mustard-Apple
Chutney
(30 g)

DESSERT
Mini Chocolate
Orange Cakes
with Ancho Chilies
(17 g)

TOTAL GRAMS OF
CARBOHYDRATES
47

Quick Meals

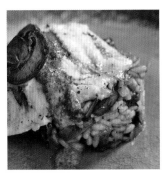

ENTRÉE
Wild Mushroom Risotto
with Seared Red Snapper
(37 g carbohydrates)

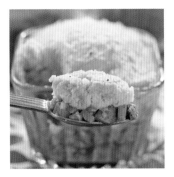

ENTRÉE
Lean
Shepherd's Pie
(40 g carbohydrates)

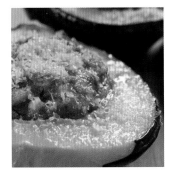

ENTRÉE
Stuffed Acorn Squash
with Chestnuts and Amaranth
(45 g carbohydrates)

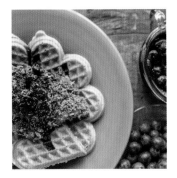

ENTRÉE
Oven Fried Chicken
and Waffles
(44 g carbohydrates)

Questions and Answers

Q: *My doctor [or nurse, or diabetes educator] told me to avoid sugar. You're telling me it's OK to have some. To whom should I listen?*

A: Your doctor or medical professional! However, you should share my principles for eating with him or her. As you know by now, I recommend consuming small amounts of sugar (aka carbohydrate) with other nutrients (such as fat, protein, and fiber) for better blood sugar control.

Q: *So I shouldn't avoid sugar?*

A: No—and it would be impossible if you tried! Most foods have some carbohydrate, which is what our bodies need for energy. If you were going to avoid all sugar, you'd never be able to eat fruits, vegetables, whole grains, or dairy (such as cheese, yogurt, and milk). So you can't avoid sugar, but when you have diabetes, you should limit how much you have.

Q: *If I should limit my sugar consumption, why do you **add more sugar** (onto the sugar that naturally exists) to your desserts?*

A: Most of the sugar we're worried about is sugar hidden in processed foods, not the sugar that's in unprocessed food. Adding only a little bit of sugar to desserts (and enjoying them in appropriate portions) is not going to cause a significant increase in your blood sugar.

Q: *What's the big deal about using artificial sweeteners?*

A: Artificial sweeteners are a processed food, and their effect in the body has not been well studied. Recent research published in a scholarly journal suggested that consuming artificial sweeteners may have negative effects on your body's ability to control blood sugar.

Q: *I've heard that fruit is high in sugar. Should I limit fruit?*

A: Fruit is higher in sugar than vegetables, but you don't need to avoid it. Just pay attention to your portion sizes, and have fruit with other foods that are high in fiber, such as nuts or seeds. Instead of having 100 percent fruit juice, have a piece of whole fruit for more fiber!

Q: *I'm on board with eating fewer carbohydrates, but it seems like they are in everything. Where should I start?*

A: Set yourself up to succeed by making small goals and tackling them one at a time. Pick a single meal or snack to start with, and decide how you will make substitutions. For instance, if you usually find yourself munching on chips from a vending machine at work as a midafternoon snack, purchase some nuts to keep in your desk (or purse) and snack on them instead. Or keep a jar of peanut butter in the office refrigerator and add one teaspoon of it to apple slices for a quick, filling treat.

Q: *I've tried eating fewer carbs and choosing healthier foods, but I don't seem to be losing any weight. Why not?*

A: Unfortunately, as much as we think we accurately remember how much we eat or how much exercise we've gotten, most people underestimate and overestimate—by a lot. So keep a record of food intake and physical activity for at least 3–5 days. Once you have a better sense of what your usual habits are, you can start making small changes more effectively.

Q: *Steamed chicken and fish are so boring. I'm sick of them! What can I do to make them tastier?*

A: When cooking using healthier methods, such as steaming or broiling, you might have to add a little flavor back in, which can also be a nice indulgence! In general, people trying to make changes to their eating patterns are more successful when they allow themselves a little indulgence, such as a small pat of butter added at the end of cooking or a small square of dark chocolate for dessert. It's all about portion control.

Q: *I eat out a lot, and now I have no idea what to order. How should I choose?*

A: First of all, you've taken a great step forward by purchasing this cookbook. One way to avoid eating out so much is to have healthy, home-cooked meals frozen and ready to go. However, if you're ordering out, try to do the following:

- Ask for sauces on the side. When you do that, *you* decide how much you eat.
- Choose half-size or lunch-size portions. Everybody knows that many restaurants serve huge portions, and if that food makes it to your plate, you're more likely to eat it.
- Choose lower-fat meals. Look for key words on menus such as "baked," "grilled," "broiled," and "steamed."
- If you're eating at the restaurant or getting take-out, refuse bread or chips.
- Don't waste calories or carbohydrates on drinks! Instead, ask for unsweetened iced tea or water with lemon.

Q: *I have a very stressful job, I get very little sleep and work too many hours to cook for myself. What options do I have left?*

A: It's tough. We all have busy lives that leave little time for "luxuries" such as spending an hour making a delicious dinner. When stressed, people tend to eat more high-calorie foods. The best thing you can do for a high-stress lifestyle is pay attention to what and how much you are eating.

Q: *Which desserts are better or worse? Are there any ones I should be avoiding?*

A: Of course not! You can have any dessert you want. Desserts are an important indulgence, but you should be careful about which ones you choose to eat. Make appropriate selections based on the nutritional content of the food. For example, your blood sugar won't rise as much if you eat fresh fruit and whipped cream as it will if you go with cake, so choose accordingly.

Q: *What is the best way to lose weight?*

A: Not all people lose weight with the same techniques or at the same rate. Nevertheless, by reducing your weight only 5 percent you can really improve your health! Start with a combination of approaches of food and physical activity. One pound of body weight equals 3,500 calories, so if you want to lose 1 pound per week, you'll need to plan on a 500-calorie deficit daily. The easiest way to do that every day is to cut out one 250-calorie snack and get 30 minutes of exercise that gets your heart rate up (even if it's only by walking).

Resources

It can be challenging to find great recipes based on the most up-to-date information for managing diabetes. Here are a few places to get started and as always, use your judgment when selecting recipes. Try to choose only those that contain real, unprocessed ingredients with appropriate portion sizes.

Academy of Nutrition and Dietetics
www.eatright.org

Diabetic Living
www.diabeticlivingonline.com

American Diabetes Association
www.diabetes.org

Mayo Clinic
www.mayoclinic.org

Acknowledgments

I would like to express my appreciation to the following people:

My family for their unconditional love and support of all my endeavors, especially my parents who have always been my greatest role models and whose strength, kindness, and positivity have pushed me to become a better person every day • Graham Burt for his time and effort to make every image better than the one before it • Jen Warner for her friendship and being one of my biggest cheerleaders • Alyson Abrami, for helping me become a seasoned recipe developer and expert at conducting cooking demonstrations • Ken Gardner, my attorney and uncle who has always been generous with his time and expertise • Diane Abrams and Christy Harrison for their effort and support years before this book was published • Jennifer Williams of Sterling Publishing, who spearheaded this project and helped the book come to fruition • And everyone at Sterling Publishing who contributed to this project.

I would also like to thank the following people: Those who provided their beautiful kitchens, props, and equipment: Peter and Lisa Gardner, Leenie and David Engel, Rob and Holly Burt, George and Connie Ongley, Sted Sweet, Karen and Gary Neems, Jimmy and Meghan Gardner, Linne Zala, Hiershenee Bhana, Kat Castro, and Matt Parola • My taste testers, for their sense of adventure, honest feedback, and support in this endeavor: Peter and Lisa Gardner, Tom Gardner and Ashley Ball, Jimmy and Meghan Gardner, Stephen and Emma Gardner, Ali and Chris Shaw, Jen Warner, Marissa Burgermaster and Ezie Cotler, Hiershenee Bhana, Linne Zala, Randal and Kelly Zala, Blake and Laurie Carr, Leigh and Tyler Lower, Andrew Vuono, Annabella and Eric Talbot, Brendan Russell and Nina Britz-Russell, and Matt Camp. •

About the Author

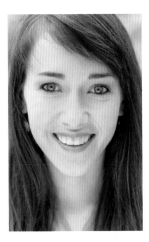

Kate Gardner, MS, RD, is a registered dietitian and culinary nutritionist specializing in whole foods and vitamins for optimal health and wellness. She received her master's degree in nutrition and exercise physiology from Columbia University, where she has been pursuing her doctorate as the first doctoral fellow of the new Laurie M. Tisch Center for Food, Education, & Policy, at Teachers College.

Prior to returning to school for her doctorate, Kate was the program coordinator for Stellar Farmers' Markets, a program run by the New York City Department of Health and Mental Hygiene, where nutrition and food professionals teach nutrition education and cooking at farmers' markets in New York City's high-need areas. Kate developed curricula and recipes and helped the program expand threefold during her tenure.

Kate's passion is improving the food environment through locally sourced food, sustainable agriculture, and the empowerment of people through education. She also enjoys counseling clients while creating individualized plans based on her clients' needs, desires, and personal goals. She currently counsels patients at her offices in Darien, Connecticut, and White Plains, New York, where she specializes in medical nutrition therapy, womens' health, and weight management in individual and group settings. Kate has consulted on various projects focused on food and sustainability. She acts as a consultant for Stone Barns Center for Food & Agriculture, the Digging Deep Campaign, and formerly for Pegasus Wellness. Kate also translates research for audiences through her personal blog, in which she dispels food and food systems myths, explains current trends in food and nutrition, and provides delicious and healthy recipes.

She has been a featured expert in print media, creates recipes for various organizations, and has hosted hundreds of cooking demonstrations. Kate has been a contributing author to New York City newspapers, the American Museum of Natural History, and *Fitness* magazine, among others.

Index